# ULTIMATE CROSS TRAINING WOD LIST
# - MORE THAN 1.000 WOD'S

BY MICHAEL SAUNDERS

## INTRODUCTION

In this book you will find hundreds of WOD'S (workouts of the day) on more than 200 pages. At first you will get lots of workouts especially designed for beginners who have never regularly trained before or haven't yet had experience with Cross Training Training.

After that there are hundreds of WOD'S just for advanced athletes. These WOD'S are divided into specific categories and eventually need equipment.

Those WOD'S cover almost every aspect of fitness training. There are WOD'S for strenght training only, WOD'S for endurance training and WOD'S that mix strenght and endurance exercises.

In addition you will get even more WOD'S that use special equipment like an AB-Wheel, a Sling Trainer (e.g. TRX System) or Jump Ropes.

In the end there is also an instruction on how to build your own WOD'S, so that you never run out of workouts.

So if you are interested in an effective and challenging training method and want to have hundreds of different workouts that will give your training variety for the next 50 years of training you've picked up the right book.


Lots of fun, success and sweat – Michael Saunders

# TABLE OF CONTENTS

Introduction ................................................................................................ 2

Table of Contents ....................................................................................... 3

What is Cross Training? ............................................................................. 6

    The goals of Cross Training ................................................................. 6

    A Cross Training session ...................................................................... 6

The WOD'S ................................................................................................. 9

    The different WOD-Categories ............................................................ 9

    What are benchmark WOD'S? ............................................................ 9

    What are hero WOD'S? ....................................................................... 9

    Structure of a WOD ............................................................................ 10

    How to use the WOD List .................................................................. 10

Total Beginner WOD'S ............................................................................. 11

    Beginner Strenght WOD'S .................................................................. 11

    Beginner Endurance WOD'S ............................................................. 33

    Beginner Strength/Endurance WOD'S .............................................. 56

Strenght only ............................................................................................ 74

    Benchmark ......................................................................................... 74

    Hero .................................................................................................... 78

    Bodyweight ........................................................................................ 95

    Free Weights .................................................................................... 103

    Kettlebell .......................................................................................... 110

- Mixed ........................................................................ 116

Endurance only ........................................................... 124
- Run ........................................................................... 124
- Swim ........................................................................ 130
- Row .......................................................................... 136
- Biking ....................................................................... 142
- Inliner ...................................................................... 148
- Endurance-Exercises ............................................... 154
- Mixed-Endurance .................................................... 159

Strenght/Endurance combined .................................. 165
- Benchmark ............................................................... 165
- Hero ......................................................................... 167
- Bodyweight .............................................................. 187
- Free Weights ............................................................ 195
- Kettlebell ................................................................. 201
- Mixed ....................................................................... 208

Other WOD'S ................................................................ 217
- Sling Trainer (e.g. TRX-Systeme) ............................. 217
- Speed Ropes ............................................................ 224
- AB-Roller ................................................................. 230
- Calisthenics Challenges .......................................... 234

Crazy WOD'S ................................................................ 238

Strenght only ..................................................................................238

   Endurance only ..............................................................................244

More Challenges ....................................................................................249

   Creating your own WOD'S ............................................................249

Links ..........................................................................................................250

Equipment ...............................................................................................250

## WHAT IS CROSS TRAINING?

Are you searching for a training method that uses elements of Gymnasitcs, Athletics, Weight Lifting, Strenght and Endurance Training? Cross Training is exactly that method. It will give you a full body workout system that uses elements from all of these sports, mixes them up and rearranges them in a special and effective way.

In Cross Training there aren't any expensive training machines necessary. Most of the time you just need a barbell and some weights. For some of the WOD'S you even need your own bodyweight only.

Cross Training is for you, if you are searching for an effective and permanently varying training system to get you in shape and challenge you individually with every workout routine.

Normally Cross Training takes place in a special gym, the so called „Box". But with this book and a little bit of experience you can train on your own, without an expensive box membership or personal trainer.

## THE GOALS OF CROSS TRAINING

Cross Training allows you to build muscle and to lose weight at the same time. The training system is organised in a way that it covers both goals. Cross Training ist primarily created to train every aspect of your fitness and when you focus on training your fitness the result will always be a healthier and fitter body.

So if you are skinny and want to gain muscle Cross Training will help you and if you are overweight and want to get ripped Cross Training will help you too.

In every Cross Training workout you will work on your strenght, endurance, coordination and flexibility. These are the factors that define fitness in general. Because of that Cross Training will challenge your fitness as a complete unit.

The beauty in it is, that every workout is individually challenging, because every workout is about pushing your individual limits.

## A CROSS TRAINING SESSION

Even though that every Cross Training workout is different, all of these follow the same structure:

1. Warm-up:

Prior to the WOD there is always a Warm-up. Because of the high intensity of the following WOD'S a warm-up is always necessary. At first you should do some light jogging, jumping jacks or high knees for 5min. Afterwards you need to warm-up your body more specificaly for the following exercises.

For example: If there are deadlifts included in the WOD you can warm yourself up by doing 3 deadlifts without any weight. Concentrate on the proper form and a slow and controlled tempo.

The Warm-up is not just for preventing injuries, it is also a good way to prepare your body for the challenges the following WOD'S include. If you warm up yourself thoughtfully and intensively before the WOD you are able to lift bigger, stronger and better. So the Warm-up will support the injury prevention and your performance.

2. Technique training

After the general and specific Warm-up you have to work on your technique. In this section of a Cross Training workout you don't have to think about bigger weights, stronger lifts and faster tempos. It is all about the proper form and the right technique.

Choose exercises that are included in the following WOD and exercises you haven't yet perfectly mastered. Use light weights and a slow tempo, till you feel more comfortable with the exercises.

3. WOD (Workout of the day)

This is the core part of every Cross Training workout. Every WOD is different und challenges you and your individual limits. They all cover different aspects of strenght, endurance, coordination and flexibility.

WOD'S aren't just workouts, they can be used as a tool to track your progress and give you important hints for your physical performance and exercise regimen.

With every WOD you get a personal benchmark. If you repeat one of the WOD's you should strive to outperform yourself and reach for better results than the last time.

4. Cool-Down

In the end of a Cross Training workout there is always a Cool-Down session. Use some light jogging, jumping jacks or high knees again und close the workout with some basic stretching exercises.

# THE WOD'S

## THE DIFFERENT WOD-CATEGORIES

The WOD'S are categorized by their main focus. This may be strenght-only, endurance-only or strenght and endurance mixed WOD'S. Within these categories the WOD'S are separated by their different exercises.

There are exercises that only need your bodyweight, others need free weights, a kettlebell or use all of these exercise-categories and mix them up. Inside the three main categories you will find these subcategories which structure the WOD'S by their specific exercises.

A strenght only WOD in the kettlebell category for example would use primarily kettlebell exercises that will train your strenght.

The WOD'S in the endurance section are divided into rowing, running, swimming, biking, bodyweight-endurance and mixed WOD'S.

After these WOD'S you will find even more WOD'S. These might need a special kind of equipment, like an AB-Whell or a Sling Trainer.

But at the beginning there are lots of WOD'S specificaly designed for beginners. You should start with these and proceed to the other ones after you have completed them.

## WHAT ARE BENCHMARK WOD'S?

Benchmark WOD'S are the most known WOD'S out there. They are named after girls and almost every Cross Training athlete knows them. Benchmark WOD'S serve as a way to track your progress and compare it to others. Try to include a benchmark WOD at least ones weekly.

## WHAT ARE HERO WOD'S?

Hero WOD'S are brutally hard, but very effective. They are named after soldiers, policemen and firemen, who died during their services. As Benchmark WOD'S Hero WOD'S are well known in the Cross Training community and can be used for tracking and comparison.

But to be honest, most of the Hero WOD'S a really hard and should only be used by advanced and well trained athletes. Hero WOD'S aren't for beginners or people who are new to Cross Training.

## STRUCTURE OF A WOD

There are mainly two kinds of WOD'S. The first („for time") needs to be completed as fast as possible. With these WOD'S you should aim for faster tempos and less or shorter resting periods.

The other kind of WOD'S is called an AMRAP WOD. AMRAP stands for „as many rounds as possible", which means that you will be given a specific time and within that time you have to complete as many rounds as you can of the exercises.

There is another sort of WOD, but it is more of a combination of the previous two. These WOD's are called „every minute on the minute" WOD'S. With every-minute-on-the-minute-WOD'S you get a workout in which you have to complete an exercise routine in every minute of the specific WOD.

## HOW TO USE THE WOD LIST

WOD'S are always constructed in the same way. At first you will see the exercises of the WOD in their order. After that you get the number of rounds to be completed or the total time the WOD will last. Finally you will be shown the goal for that WOD. Sometimes it's an every-minute-on-the-minute-WOD, sometimes an AMRAP, but most of the time it is all about completing the WOD as fast as you can („for time").

## TOTAL BEGINNER WOD'S

If you have never before used a workout routine for a longer period of time or if you're totally new to Cross Training you should consider using the total beginner WOD'S first.

With these WOD'S you will get a good starting point which will be challenging, but not to much challenging. The WOD'S will give you a good basis for the upcoming Benchmark and Hero WOD'S and will teach you the necessary exercises and structures in a fashion specificaly designed for beginners.

## BEGINNER STRENGHT WOD'S

# **Bodyweight**

„BS1"

- 15 Squats
- Maximum Pull-ups

5 rounds
For time or maximum repetitions

„BS2"

- Maximum Push-ups
- 90s Rest

5 rounds
Maximum repetitions

„BS3"

- 10 Squats

- 10 Push-ups

5 rounds
For time

## „BS4"

- 5 Push-ups
- 5 Pull-ups
- 10 Squats

AMRAP: As many rounds as possible in 10min

## „BS5"

- 100m Lunge
- 60s Rest

3 rounds
For time

## „BS6"

- Maximum Push-ups
- Maximum Pull-ups
- 90s Rest

3 rounds
Maximum repetitions

## „BS7"

- 50 Squats
- 25 Push-ups
- 10 Pull-ups

For time

## „BS8"

- Maximum Jump Squats
- 50 Double unders
- 60s Rest

3 rounds
Maximum repetitions of Push-ups

## „BS9"

100 Crunches

For time

## „BS10"

- 5min Lunges
- 5min Squats

Maximum repetitions

## „BS11"

- 10 Push-ups
- 15 Squats

- 20 Crunches

3 rounds
For time

## „BS12"

- 10 Crunches
- 5 Push-ups
- 3 Pull-ups

5 rounds
For time

## „BS13"

- 10 Box Jumps
- 5 Pull-ups

7 rounds
For time

## „BS14"

- 20 Crunches
- 20 Lunges
- 60s Rest

5 rounds
For time

## „BS15"

- 2 Box Jumps
- 2 Push-ups
- 2 Crunches

AMRAP: As many rounds as possible in 8min

## „BS16"

- 20s Squats
- 10s Rest

8 rounds
Maximum repetitions

## „BS17"

- 20s Push-ups
- 10s Rest

8 rounds
Maximum repetitions

## „BS18"

- 20s Crunches
- 10s Rest

8 rounds
Maximum repetitions

„BS19"

- 1 Push-up
- 1 Crunch

Every minute one more repetition, till you can't do the necessary number of repetitions per exercise

„BS20"

- 10 Pull-ups
- 20 Push-ups
- 30 Crunches
- 40 Squats

For time

## **Free Weights (Barbell) – Use light weights**

„BS21"

- 10 Squats
- 60s Rest

3 rounds
For time

„BS22"

- 20 Benchpress
- 90s Rest

3 rounds
For time

## „BS23"

- 10 Row
- 10 Squats
- 30s Rest

5 rounds
For time

## „BS24"

- 20 Row
- 20 Benchpress
- 20 Squats
- 20 Lunge

For time

## „BS25"

- 10 Power clean
- 10 Squats
- 60s Rest

4 rounds
For time

## „BS26"

- 20 Deadlift
- 20 Benchpress
- 20 Squats
- 20 Push press

For time

## „BS27"

- 5 Push Press
- 5 Overhead Squats
- 5 Power clean

AMRAP: As many rounds as possible in 8min

## „BS28"

- 25 Sumo Deadlift
- 25 Benchpress

2 rounds
For time

## „BS29"

- 50 Overhead Lunges
- 50 Overhead Squats

For time

## „BS30"

100 Benchpress

For time

## „BS31"

- 1 Benchpress
- 1 Row
- 1 Deadlift

Every minute one more repetition, till you can't do the necessary number of repetitions per exercise

## „BS32"

Sumo Deadlift

21-15-9 Repetitions
For time

## „BS33"

- 3 Clean and Jerk
- 5 Deadlift
- 3 Front Squat

5 rounds
For time

## „BS34"

1 Push jerk

Every minute one more repetition, till you can't do the necessary number of repetitions per exercise

## "BS35"

- Deadlift
- Benchpress

10-8-6-4-2 Repetitions
For time

## "BS36"

- 10 Backwards Lunge
- 10 Forward Lunge
- 60s Rest

5 rounds
For time

## "BS37"

5 Benchpress

5 rounds, heavier weights every round

## "BS38"

- 30 Row
- 20 Overhead Squat
- 10 Benchpress

2 rounds
For time

---

„BS39"

Clean to Thruster

Technique only (do minimum 100 repetitions with light weights)

---

„BS40"

100 Push Press

For time

# Kettlebell (use a kettlebell with every exercise – use light weights)

„BS41"

- 10 Snatch
- 10 Press
- 90s Rest

3 rounds
For time

---

„BS42"

Swing

Technique only (do minimum 100 repetitions with light weights)

## „BS43"

- 30 Clean and Jerk
- 30 Swing

For time

## „BS44"

- Swing
- Push-up

21-12-9 Repetitions
For time

## „BS45"

- 5 Sumo Deadlift
- 5 Press
- 5 Swing
- 60s Rest

3 rounds
For time

## „BS46"

Thruster

Technique only (do minimum 100 repetitions with light weights)

## „BS47"

- 10 Clean
- 10 Thruster
- 10 Windmill
- 60s Rest

3 rounds
For time

## „BS48"

- 20s Snatch
- 10s Rest

8 rounds
Maximum repetitions

## „BS49"

1 Thruster

Every minute one more repetition, till you can't do the necessary number of repetitions per exercise

## „BS50"

Double clean

1-2-3-4-5-6-7-8 Repetitions
For time

# Mixed (Bodyweight, free Weights and Kettlebell combined)

Use kettlebells only, if they are explicitly mentioned, use free weights if you ain't got a kettlebell

## „BS51"

- Deadlift
- Thruster

21-15-9 Repetitions
For time

## „BS52"

- 9 Power Snatch
- 15 Wall ball

2 rounds
For time

## „BS53"

- Thrusters
- Weighted Pull-ups

15-12-9 Repetitions
For time

## „BS54"

- 30 Overhead Squats
- 10 Pull-ups

For time

## „BS55"

- Power clean
- Ring Dips

12-8-4 Repetitions
For time

## „BS56"

- 3 Deadlift
- 15 Wall ball

5 rounds
For time

## „BS57"

- 20s Hang Power clean
- 10s Rest
- 20s Kettlebell Push Press
- 10s Rest

4 rounds
Maximum repetitions

## „BS58"

- Sumo Deadlift
- Box Jump

21-12-5 Repetitions
For time

## „BS59"

- 20 Pull-ups
- 40 Kettlebell Swing

For time

## „BS60"

- 20 Ball Slam
- 20 Push-ups
- 20 Crunches

2 rounds
For time

## „BS61"

- 15 Front Squat
- 25 Kettlebell Swings
- 30 Crunches

2 rounds
For time

## „BS62"

- 6 Sumo Deadlift
- 6 Power Snatch
- 6 Pull-ups

AMRAP: As many rounds as possible in 8min

## „BS63"

- 7 Back Squats
- 7 Pull-ups
- 7 Benchpress

3 rounds
For time

## „BS64"

- 20 Ball Slams
- 25 Box Jumps
- 30 Kettlebell Press

For time

## „BS65"

- 1 Row
- 1 Push-up
- 1 Kettlebell Swing

Every minute one more repetition, till you can't do the necessary number of repetitions per exercise

„BS66"

- 20 Squats
- 20 Benchpress
- 20 Crunches

3 rounds
For time


„BS67"

- 5 Deadlift
- 8 Push Press
- 10 Pull-ups

2 rounds
For time


„BS68"

- 10 Deadlift
- 10 Kettlebell Swing
- 10 Push-ups

3 rounds
For time


„BS69"

- Back Squat
- Push-ups

- Kettlebell Swing

21-12-6 Repetitions
For time

## „BS70"

- 30s Benchpress
- 10s Rest
- 30s Push-ups
- 10s Rest

3 rounds
Maximum repetitions

## „BS71"

- 45s Box Jumps
- 15s Rest
- 45s Deadlift
- 15s Rest
- 45s Squats
- 15s Rest

3 rounds
For time

## „BS72"

- 20 Push-ups
- 10 Pull-ups
- 5 Kettlebell Swings

3 rounds
For time

„BS73"

- 25 Box Jumps
- 20 Kettlebell Swings
- 15 Push-ups
- 10 Overhead Squats
- 5 Push Press

2 rounds
For time

„BS74"

Pistol Squat Training

Technique only, try to go deeper with every set

„BS75"

- 5 Deadlift
- 5 Benchpress
- 5 Pull-ups

3 rounds
For time

„BS76"

- 30 Double unders
- 30 Crunches

5 rounds
For time

## „BS77"

- 1 Lunge (each leg)
- 1 Kettlebell Wing
- 1 Pull-up

Every minute one more repetition, till you can't do the necessary number of repetitions per exercise

## „BS78"

- 3 Power Snatches
- 3 Pull-ups
- 6 Push-ups
- 9 Box Jumps

AMRAP: As many rounds as possible in 8min

## „BS79"

- Power Snatch
- Box Jumps
- Kettlebell Thruster

3 rounds
Maximum repetitions for every exercise

„BS80"

- 8 Kettlebell Thruster
- 8 Pull-ups
- 8 Benchpress

3 rounds
For time

## BEGINNER ENDURANCE WOD'S

# **Running**

„BE1"

- 1min Run
- 1min Walk

10 rounds
Maximum distance


„BE2"

- 1min Run
- 1min Walk

15 rounds
Maximum distance


„BE3"

- 1min Run
- 1min Walk

20 rounds
Maximum distance


„BE4"

- 2min Run
- 1min Walk

10 rounds
Maximum distance

## „BE5"

- 5min Run
- 1min Walk

5 rounds
Maximum distance

## „BE6"

- 10min Run
- 1min Walk

3 rounds
Maximum distance

## „BE7"

30min Run

Maximum distance

## „BE8"

- 20s Sprint
- 20s Rest

4 rounds
Maximum distance

## „BE9"

- 20s Sprint
- 10s Rest

8 rounds
Maximum distance

## „BE10"

1000m Run

For time

## „BE11"

- 100m Run
- 25m Sprint
- 75m Walk

4 rounds
For time

## „BE12"

- 10m Sprint
- 90m Walk
- 20m Sprint
- 80m Walk
- 40m Sprint
- 60m Walk

- 80m Sprint
- 20m Walk
- 100m Sprint

For time

## „BE13"

- 200m Run
- 30s Rest

8 rounds
For time

## „BE14"

- 400m Run
- 100m Sprint
- 100m Walk
- 100m Sprint
- 100m Walk

2 rounds
For time

## „BE15"

2500m Run

For time

## „BE16"

- 400m Run
- 3min Rest

4 rounds
For time

## „BE17"

10m Sprint

Every minute plus 10m, till you can't run the distance in minute

## „BE18"

- 400m Run
- 1min Rest
- 200m Sprint
- 1min Rest
- 100m Sprint
- 1min Rest
- 50m Sprint
- 1min Rest
- 25m Sprint

For time

## „BE19"

5000m Run

For time

„BE20"

45min Run without a rest

Maximum distance

# **Swimming**

„BE21"

- 1min Breaststroke (Technique)
- 1min Rest

8 rounds

„BE22"

- 1min Freestyle (Technique)
- 1min Rest

8 rounds

„BE23"

- 1min Backstroke (Technique)
- 1min Rest

8 rounds

„BE24"

- 1min Butterfly (Technique)
- 1min Rest

8 rounds

„BE25"

- 2min Breaststroke (Technique)
- 1min Rest

8 rounds

## „BE26"

- 2min Breaststroke
- 1min Freestyle
- 1min Rest

4 rounds
Maximum distance

## „BE27"

- 25m Backstroke
- 30s Rest
- 25m Freestyle
- 30s Rest
- 25m Breaststroke
- 30s Rest

4 rounds
For time

## „BE28"

200m Swim without a rest

For time

## „BE29"

10min Swim without a rest

Maximum distance

## „BE30"

15min Freestyle without a rest

Maximum distance

# Biking

**„BE31"**

- 10min Bike
- 2min Rest

2 rounds
Maximum distance

**„BE32"**

- 15min Bike
- 2min Rest

2 rounds
Maximum distance

**„BE33"**

5000m Bike

For time

**„BE34"**

- 20min Bike
- 1min Rest

2 rounds
Maximum distance

„BE35"

10.000m Bike

For time

„BE36"

- 1000m Bike
- 100m Bike – Sprint

4 rounds
For time

„BE37"

- 20s Bike – Sprint
- 10s Rest

4 rounds
Maximum distance

„BE38"

- 1min Bike
- 20s Bike – Sprint
- 10s Rest

4 rounds
Maximum distance

„BE39"

10m Bike – Sprint

Every minute plus 10m, till you can't do the distance in one minute. The rest of every minute is a just a rollout.

"BE40"

- 90m Bike
- 10m Bike – Sprint

8 rounds
For time

## **Endurance-Exercises**

"BE41"

- 5min Burpee (Technique – slow tempo)
- 2min Rest

2 rounds

"BE42"

- 5min Jumping Jack (Technique – slow tempo)
- 2min Rest

2 rounds

"BE43"

- 5min High knees (Technique – slow tempo)

- 2min Rest

2 rounds

## „BE44"

- 10 Burpees
- 20 Jumping Jacks
- 1min Rest

3 rounds
For time

## „BE45"

- 5 Burpees
- 10 Jumping Jacks
- 3min Rest

5 rounds
For time

## „BE46"

1 Burpee

Every minute one repetition more, till you reach 6 repetitions

## „BE47"

2 Jumping Jacks

Every minute two repetitions more, till you reach 20 repetitions

### „BE48"

- 2min High knees
- 2min Rest

3 rounds
Maximum repetitions

### „BE49"

- 20s Jumping Jacks
- 10s Rest

4 rounds
Maximum repetitions

### „BE50"

- 10s Burpee
- 20s Rest
- 10s High knees
- 20s Rest

3 rounds
Maximum repetitions

# **Row**

### „BE51"

- 100m Row
- 100m Rest

5 rounds
For time

### „BE52"

- 2min Row
- 1min Rest

3 rounds
Maximum distance

### „BE53"

- 5min Row
- 1min Rest

2 rounds
For time

### „BE54"

- 100kcal Row
- 1min Rest

3 rounds
For time

## „BE55"

1000m Row

For time

## „BE56"

10min Row

Maximum distance

## „BE57"

- 20s Row – Sprint
- 40s Row (slowly)

3 rounds
Maximum distance

## „BE58"

- 5min Row
- 1min Rest

5 rounds
Maximum distance

## „BE59"

10m Row

Every minute plus 10m, till you can't do the distance in one minute

---

„BE60"

2500m Row

For time

# Mixed Endurance Exercises

„BE61"

- 1min Run
- 5 Burpees
- 2min Rest

5 rounds
For time


„BE62"

- 1min Run
- 5 Burpees
- 1min Rest

5 rounds
For time


„BE63"

- 1min Run
- 10 Jumping Jacks
- 2min Rest

5 rounds
For time


„BE64"

- 2min Run
- 20 High knees

- 2min Rest

5 rounds
For time

## „BE65"

- 20s Run - Sprint
- 5 Burpees
- 10 Jumping Jacks
- 2min Rest

3 rounds
For time

## „BE66"

- 50m Swim (Freestyle)
- 20 Jumping Jacks

4 rounds
For time

## „BE67"

- 5min Run
- 1min High knees

3 rounds
Maximum distance and repetitions

## „BE68"

- 100m Swim (Breaststroke)
- 10 Burpees

3 rounds
For time

## „BE69"

- 10min Run
- 10min Bike
- 20 Burpees

Maximum distance and tempo

## „BE70"

- 10 Burpees
- 20 Jumping Jacks
- 50m Sprint

2 rounds
For time

## „BE71"

- 1min Row
- 1min High knees

3 rounds
Maximum distance and repetitions

## „BE72"

- 3min Bike
- 20s Sprint
- 20s Rest
- 20s Sprint (back)

3 rounds
Maximum distance

## „BE73"

- 1 Burpee
- 10m Sprint

Every minute plus one repetition and 10m, till you can't do the reps or distance in one minute

## „BE74"

- 1 Burpee
- 1 High knees
- 1 Jumping Jacks
- 10m Sprint

AMRAP: As many rounds as possible in 10min

## „BE75"

- 100 Rope Jumps (Double Jump)
- 1000m Run

For time

## „BE76"

- 50 Jumping Jacks
- 50m Sprint

3 rounds
For time

## „BE77"

- 5min Bike
- 10 Burpees

4 rounds
Maximum distance by bike and Burpees for time

## „BE78"

- 50kcal Row
- 50kcal Bike

4 rounds
For time

## „BE79"

- 100m Swim (Freestyle)
- 1000m Run
- 3000m Bike

For time

## „BE80"

- 4 Burpee
- 10 High knees
- 10 Jumping Jacks
- 100m Sprint

AMRAP: As many rounds as possible in 10min

## BEGINNER STRENGTH/ENDURANCE WOD'S

## **Bodyweight**

„BSE1"

- Push-ups
- Jump Squats
- Burpees

15-8-4 Repetitions
For time

„BSE2"

- 15 Squats
- 10 Push-ups
- 5 Pull-ups

AMRAP: As many rounds as possible in 6min

„BSE3"

- 10 Push-ups
- 400m Run

4 rounds
For time

„BSE4"

- 30 Crunches

- 30 Jumping Jacks

5 rounds
For time

## „BSE5"

- 20s Squats
- 10s Rest
- 20s Sprint
- 10s Rest

3 rounds
Maximum repetitions and distance

## „BSE6"

- 5 Box Jumps
- 5 Push-ups
- 10 High knees

3 rounds
For time

## „BSE7"

- 100m Run-Sprint
- 5 Push-ups

5 rounds
For time

## „BSE8"

- 50 Push-ups
- 2500m Run

Just finish it
For time

## „BSE9"

- 100 Crunches
- 100 Jumping Jacks

For time

## „BSE10"

- 10 Pull-ups
- 20 Push-ups
- 40 Air Squats
- 100 High knees

For time

## „BSE11"

- 15 Box Jumps
- 400m Run

2 rounds
For time

## „BSE12"

- 33 Squats
- 33 Crunches
- 1000m Run

For time

## „BSE13"

- 5 Burpees
- 5 Push-ups
- 5 High knees
- 5 Squats
- 5 Jumping Jacks
- 5 Crunches

3 rounds
For time

## „BSE14"

1000m Run

Every 100m 10 Squats
For time

## „BSE15"

- 50m Swim (Freestyle)
- 5 Squats
- 5 Push-ups

4 rounds
For time

## „BSE16"

- 20 Rope Jumps (Double Jump)
- 10 Crunches

5 rounds
For time

## „BSE17"

- 10m Run-Sprint
- 5 Burpees
- 5 Squats

3 rounds
For time

## „BSE18"

- 10 Pull-ups
- 20 Burpees
- 40 Squats

For time

## „BSE19"

- 100m Bike-Sprint

- 5 Push-ups

5 rounds
For time

## „BSE20"

- 1000m Run
- 10 Squats
- 800m Run
- 10 Squats
- 400m
- 10 Squats
- 200m Run
- 10 Squats
- 100m Run

For time

# Free Weights – Use light weights

„BSE21"

- 10 Benchpress
- 10 Squat
- 1000m Run

For time

„BSE22"

- 10 Row
- 10 Push Press
- 400m Run

2 rounds
For time

„BSE23"

- 50 Burpees
- 50 Deadlift

For time

„BSE24"

- 5 Row
- 100m Sprint

5 rounds
For time

## „BSE25"

- 1min Push Press
- 1min Squat
- 1min Jumping Jack
- 1min Rest

2 rounds
Maximum repetitions

## „BSE26"

- 5 Deadlift
- 5 Burpee
- 5 Lunge

AMRAP: As many rounds as possible in 8min

## „BSE27"

- 50 Push Press
- 50 Burpees

For time

## „BSE28"

- 25 Benchpress
- 25 Row
- 3000m Bike

For time

## „BSE29"

- 50 Clean
- 1000m Run

For time

## „BSE30"

- 1 Row
- 1 Squat
- 1 Burpee

Every minute plus one repetition, till you can't do the reps in one minute

## „BSE31"

- 5 Deadlift
- 5 Push Press
- 100m Run-Sprint

3 rounds
For time

## „BSE32"

- 25 Row
- 25 Snatch
- 100 Jumping Jacks

For time

---

„BSE33"

- 20 Benchpress
- 20 Deadlift
- 20 Push Press
- 5000m Run

For time

---

„BSE34"

- 10 Benchpress
- 100m Sprint
- 10 Clean
- 100m Sprint

4 rounds
For time

---

„BSE35"

- 50 Snatch
- 150 Jumping Jacks

For time

---

„BSE36"

- 400m Run

- 10 Row

4 rounds
For time

## „BSE37"

- 5 Burpee
- 5 Overhead Squat
- 5 Burpee
- 5 Squat
- 5 Burpee
- 5 Lunge

2 rounds
For time

## „BSE38"

Row is the endurance exercise

- 50kcal Row
- 20 Deadlift
- 50kcal Row
- 20 Clean
- 50kcal Row
- 20 Squat

2 rounds
For time

## „BSE39"

- 100 Benchpress
- 250 High knees

For time

## „BSE40"

- 1 Benchpress
- 1 Squat
- 1 Burpee

Every minute plus one repetition, till you can't do the reps in one minute

## **Kettlebell (Use light weights and focus on technique)**

**„BSE41"**

- 5 Swing
- 400m Run

4 rounds
For time

**„BSE42"**

- 10 Clean
- 10 Windmill
- 10 Burpees

2 rounds
For time

**„BSE43"**

- 5 Press
- 5 Clean
- 25 Jumping Jacks

2 rounds
For time

**„BSE44"**

- 50 Double Snatch
- 1000m Run

For time

## „BSE45"

- 4 Swings
- 4 Burpees
- 4 Clean and Jerk

AMRAP: As many rounds as possible in 8min

## „BSE46"

- 4 Burpees
- 4 Squats
- 4 Burpees
- 4 Swings
- 1min Rest

4 rounds
For time

## „BSE47"

- 10 Push-ups
- 10 Swings
- 10 Clean
- 10 Squats
- 100m Sprint

For time

## „BSE48"

- 1 Clean and Jerk
- 1 Squat
- 1 Burpee

Every minute plus one repetition, till you can't do the reps in one minute

## „BSE49"

Row is the endurance exercise

- 50kcal Row
- 5 Swing
- 50kcal Row
- 5 Clean

2 rounds
For time

## „BSE50"

- 50 Snatch
- 800m Run

For time

# Mixed

Use free weights and bodyweight exercises if kettlebells and other equipment ist not explicitly mentioned

### „BSE51"

- 5 Benchpress
- 5 Pull-ups
- 5 Burpees

3 rounds
For time

### „BSE52"

- 10 Kettlebell Swing
- 10 Deadlift
- 25 Jumping Jacks

2 rounds
For time

### „BSE53"

- 100m Sprint
- 5 Push-ups
- 100m Sprint
- 5 Squats
- 100m Sprint
- 5 Crunches
- 100m Sprint
- 5 Kettlebell Clean and Jerk

For time

## „BSE54"

- 5 Benchpress
- 10 High knees
- 5 Squats

AMRAP: As many rounds as possible in 8min

## „BSE55"

- Thruster
- Pull-ups
- Burpee

12-6-2 Repetitions
For time

## „BSE56"

- 3 Deadlift
- 5 Box Jumps
- 8 Jumping Jacks

4 rounds
For time

## „BSE57"

- 1min Benchpress
- 1min Kettlebell Swing
- 1min High knees

- 1min Rest

2 rounds
Maximum repetitions

## „BSE58"

- 50 Benchpress
- 50 Kettlebell Squats
- 50 Jumping Jacks

For time

## „BSE59"

- 5 Pull-ups
- 25 Double unders
- 10 Lunge
- 1000m Sprint

For time

## „BSE60"

Row is the endurance exercise

- 50kcal Row
- 5 Back Squats
- 50kcal Row
- 5 Kettlebell Thruster

2 rounds
For time

## STRENGHT ONLY

You will find the more advanced WOD'S here. If you've just started working out regularly i recommend starting with the Beginner WOD'S in the last chapter.

## BENCHMARK

### „ANGIE"

- 100 Pull-ups
- 100 Push-ups
- 100 Sit-ups
- 100 Squats

For time
Do all repetitions of an exercise before moving on to the next one

### „BARBARA"

- 20 Pull-ups
- 30 Push-ups
- 40 Sit-ups
- 50 Squats

5 rounds
For time

### „CHELSEA"

- 5 Pull-ups
- 10 Push-ups
- 15 Squats

Every minute for 30min in total

## „CINDY"

- 5 Pull-ups
- 10 Push-ups
- 15 Squats

AMRAP: As Many Rounds As Possible in 20min

## „DIANE"

- Deadlift 225lbs (ca. 100kg)
- Handstand Push-ups

21-15-9 Repetitions
For time

## „ELIZABETH"

- Clean 135lbs (ca. 60kg)
- Ring Dips

21-15-9 Repetitions
For time

## „FRAN"

- Thruster 95lbs (ca. 40kg)
- Pull-ups

21-15-9 Repetitions
For time

## „GRACE"

- Clean and Jerk 135lbs (ca. 60kg)

30 Repetitions for time

## „ISABEL"

- Snatch 135lbs (ca. 60kg)

30 Repetitions for time

## „KAREN"

- 150 Wallball 20lbs (ca. 8kg)

For time

## „LINDA" (AKA "3 BARS OF DEATH")

- Deadlift 1.5x Bodyweight
- Benchpress Bodyweight
- Clean 0.75x Bodyweight

10/9/8/7/6/5/4/3/2/1 Repetitions per round
For time

## „MARY"

- 5 Handstand Push-ups
- 10 One-Legged Squats (Pistols)
- 15 Pull-ups

AMRAP: As Many Rounds As Possible in 20min

## „ANNIE"

- Double Unders
- Sit-ups

50-40-30-20-10 Repetitions per round
For time

## „LYNNE"

- Benchpress Bodyweight
- Pull-ups

5 rounds
Maximum repetitions

# HERO

## „JT"

- Handstand Push-ups
- Ring Dips
- Push-ups

21-15-9 Repetitions
For time

## „JOSH"

- 21 Overhead Squats 95lbs (ca. 40kg)
- 42 Pull-ups
- 15 Overhead Squats 95lbs (ca. 40kg)
- 30 Pull-ups
- 9 Overhead Squats 95lbss (ca. 40kg)
- 18 Pull-ups

For time

## „JASON"

- 100 Squats
- 5 Muscle-ups
- 75 Squats
- 10 Muscle-ups
- 50 Squats
- 15 Muscle-ups
- 25 Squats
- 20 Muscle-ups

For time

## „JOSHIE"

- 21 Dumbbell Snatch 40lbs (ca. 15kg) right arm
- 21 L Pull-ups
- 21 Dumbbell Snatch 40lbs (ca. 15kg) left arm
- 21 L Pull-ups

Snatches are full Snatches
3 rounds
For time

## „NATE"

- 2 Muscle-ups
- 4 Handstand Push-ups
- 8 Kettlebell Swings 2 pood (apx 72lbs – ca. 30kg)

AMRAP: As Many Rounds As Possible in 20min

## „RANDY"

- 75 Power Snatch 75lbs (ca. 35kg)

For time

## „TOMMY V"

(ft = feet – 15ft = ca. 4,5m)

- 21 Thrusters 115lbs (ca. 50kg)
- 15 ft Rope Climb, 12 Ascends
- 15 Thrusters 115lbs (ca. 50kg)

- 15 ft Rope Climb, 9 Ascends
- 9 Thrusters 115lbs (ca. 50kg)
- 15 ft Rope Climb, 6 Ascends

For time

## „ERIN"

- 15 Dumbbells Split Clean 40lbs (ca. 15kg)
- 21 Pull-ups

5 rounds
For time

## „DT"

- 12 Deadlift 155lbs (ca. 70kg)
- 9 Hang Power Clean 155lbs (ca. 70kg)
- 6 Push Jerk 155lbs (ca. 70kg)

5 rounds
For time

## „DANNY"

- 30 Box Jump 24"
- 20 Push Press 115lbs (ca. 50kg)
- 30 Pull-ups

AMRAP: As Many Rounds As Possible in 20min

## „HANSEN"

- 30 Kettlebell Swing 2 pood (apx 70lbs – ca. 30kg)
- 30 Burpees
- 30 Glute-Ham Sit-ups

5 rounds
For time

## „TYLER"

- 7 Muscle-ups
- 21 Sumo-Deadlift High-Pull 95lbs (ca. 40kg)

5 rounds
For time

## „STEPHEN"

- Glute-Ham Sit-ups
- Back Extensions
- Knees to Elbow
- Stiff Legged Deadlift 95lbs (ca. 45kg)

30-25-20-15-10-5 Repetitions for all exercises

## „GARRETT"

- 75 Squats
- 25 Ring Handstand Push-ups
- 25 L Pull-ups

3 rounds
For time

## „WAR FRANK"

- 25 Muscle-ups
- 100 Squats
- 35 Glute-Ham Sit-ups

3 rounds
For time

## „MCGHEE"

- 5 Deadlift 275lbs (ca. 125kg)
- 13 Push-ups
- 9 Box Jumps 24" Box

AMRAP: As Many Rounds As Possible in 20min

## „PAUL"

- 50 Double Unders
- 35 Knees to Elbows
- Overhead Walk 20 yards 185lbs (ca. 85kg)

5 rounds
For time

## „ARNIE"

With a single 2 pood kettlebell (apx 72lbs – ca. 30kg):

- 21 Turkish get-ups, Right arm
- 50 Kettlebell Swings
- 21 Overhead squats, Left arm
- 50 Kettlebell Swings

- 21 Overhead squats, Right arm
- 50 Kettlebell Swings
- 21 Turkish get-ups, Left arm

For time

## „JOHNSON"

- 9 Deadlift 245lbs (ca. 115kg)
- 8 Muscle-ups
- 9 Squat Clean 155lbs (ca. 70kg)

AMRAP: As Many Rounds As Possible in 20min

## „ROY"

- 15 Deadlift 225lbs (ca. 100kg)
- 20 Box Jumps 24" Box
- 25 Pull-ups

5 rounds
For time

## „ADAM BROWN"

- 24 Deadlift 295lbs (ca. 140kg)
- 24 Box Jumps, 24" Box
- 24 Wallball 20lbs (ca. 8kg)
- 24 Bench Press 195lbs (ca. 90kg)
- 24 Box Jumps 24" Box
- 24 Wallball 20lbs (ca. 8kg)
- 24 Clean 145lbs (ca. 65kg)

2 rounds
For time

## „COE"

- 10 Thruster 65lbs (ca. 30kg)
- 10 Ring Push-ups

10 rounds
For time

## „JACK"

- 10 Push press 115lbs (ca. 50kg)
- 10 Kettlebell Swings 1.5 pood (apx. 55lbs – ca. 25kg)
- 10 Box jumps 24" Box

AMRAP: As Many Rounds As Possible in 20min

## „BLAKE"

- 100 ft Walking lunge mit 45lb plate (ca. 20kg) Overhead
- 30 Box jump 24" Box
- 20 Wallball shots 20lb (ca. 8kg)
- 10 Handstand push-ups

4 rounds
For time

## „THOMPSON"

- 15 ft (ca. 4,5m) Rope Climb, 1 Ascends (Starting point: seated on the floor)
- 29 Back Squat 95lbs (ca. 40kg)
- 10m Barbell Farmer carry 135lbs (ca. 60kg)

10 rounds
For time

## „LEDESMA"

- 5 Parallette Handstand Push-ups
- 10 Toes through Rings
- 15 Medicine Ball Cleans 20lbs (ca. 8kg)

AMRAP: As Many Rounds As Possible in 20min

## „WITTMAN"

- 15 Kettlebell Swings 1.5 pood (apx. 55lbs – ca. 20kg)
- 15 Power Clean (M=95lbs – ca. 40kg, F=65lbs – ca. 30kg)
- 15 Box Jumps (M=24", F=18")

7 rounds
For time

## „WEAVER"

- 10 L Pull-ups
- 15 Push-ups
- 15 Chest to bar Pull-ups
- 15 Push-ups
- 20 Pull-ups
- 15 Push-ups

4 rounds
For time

## „HAMMER"

M=135lbs – ca. 60kg; F=95lbs – ca. 40kg)

- 5 Power Clean (M=135lbs. F=95lbs)
- 10 Front Squat (M=135lbs. F=95lbs)
- 5 Jerk (M=135lbs. F=95lbs)
- 20 Pull-ups
- 90s Rest

5 rounds
For time

## „WILMOT"

- 50 Squats
- 25 Ring dips

6 rounds
For time

## „MORRISON"

- Wallballs
- Box jump 24"
- Kettlebell Swings 1.5 pood (apx 55lbs – ca. 20kg)

50-40-30-20-10 Repetitions
For time

## „GATOR"

- 5 Front Squat 185lbs (ca. 85kg)
- 26 Ring Push-ups

8 rounds
For time

## „MEADOWS"

- 20 Muscle-ups
- 25 Lowers from an inverted hang on the rings, slowly, with straight body and arms
- 30 Ring Handstand Push-ups
- 35 Ring Rows
- 40 Ring Push-ups

For time

## „SANTIAGO"

- 18 Hang Squat Clean 35lb Dumbbells (ca. 20kg)
- 18 Pull-ups
- 10 Power Clean (M=135lbs –ca. 60kg, F=95lbs – ca. 40kg)
- 10 Handstand Push-ups

7 rounds
For time

## „CARSE"

- Squat Clean (M=95lbs – ca. 40kg, F=65lbs – ca. 30kg)
- Double unders

- Deadlift 185lbs (ca. 85kg)
- Box jump 24"

21-18-15-12-9-6-3 Repetitions
For time

## „BRADSHAW"

- 3 Handstand Push-ups
- 6 Deadlift 225lbs (ca. 100kg)
- 12 Pull-ups
- 24 Double unders

10 rounds
For time

## „RICKY"

- 10 Pull-ups
- 5 Deadlift 75lb (ca. 30kg) Dumbbells
- 8 Push Press (M=135lbs – ca. 60kg, F=95lbs – ca. 40kg)

AMRAP: As Many Rounds As Possible in 20min

## „ZIMMERMAN"

- 11 Chest to Bar Pull-ups
- 2 Deadlifts 315lbs (ca. 150kg)
- 10 Handstand Push-ups

AMRAP: As Many Rounds As Possible in 25min

## „PHEEZY"

- 5 Front Squat 165lbs (ca. 75kg)
- 18 Pull-ups
- 5 Deadlift 225lbs (ca. 100kg)
- 18 Toes to Bar
- 5 Push Jerk 165lbs (ca. 75kg)
- 18 Hand Release Push-ups

3 rounds
For time


## „J.J"

- 1 Squat Clean 185lbs (ca. 85kg)
- 10 Parallette Handstand Push-ups
- 2 Squat Clean 185lbs (ca. 85kg)
- 9 Parallette Handstand Push-ups
- 3 Squat Clean 185lbs (ca. 85kg)
- 8 Parallette Handstand Push-ups
- 4 Squat Clean 185lbs (ca. 85kg)
- 7 Parallette Handstand Push-ups
- 5 Squat Clean 185lbs (ca. 85kg)
- 6 Parallette Handstand Push-ups
- 6 Squat Clean 185lbs (ca. 85kg)
- 5 Parallette Handstand Push-ups
- 7 Squat Clean 185lbs (ca. 85kg)
- 4 Parallette Handstand Push-ups
- 8 Squat Clean 185lbs (ca. 85kg)
- 3 Parallette Handstand Push-ups
- 9 Squat Clean 185lbs (ca. 85kg)
- 2 Parallette Handstand Push-ups
- 10 Squat Clean 185lbs (ca. 85kg)
- 1 Parallette Handstand Push-ups

For time

## „BRIAN"

- 15 ft (ca. 4,5m) Rope Climb 5 Ascends
- 25 Back Squat 185lbs (ca. 85kg)

3 rounds
For time

## „NICK"

- 10 Hang Squat Clean 45 pound (ca. 20kg) Dumbbells
- 6 Handstand Push-ups on Dumbbells

12 rounds
For time

## „SHIP"

- 7 Squat Clean 185lbs (ca. 85kg)
- 8 Burpee Box Jumps, 36"

9 rounds
For time

## „HOLLEYMAN"

- 5 Wallballs
- 3 Handstand Push-ups
- 1 Power Clean 225lbs (ca. 100kg)

30 rounds
For time

## „ADRIAN"

- 3 Forward Rolls
- 5 Wall Climbs
- 7 Toes to Bar 9 Box Jumps 30"

7 rounds
For time

## „TOM"

- 7 Muscle-ups
- 11 Thruster 155lbs (ca. 70kg)
- 14 Toes to Bar

AMRAP: As Many Rounds As Possible in 20min

## „SEAN"

- 11 Chest to Bar Pull-ups
- 22 Front Squat (M=75lbs – ca. 30kg, F=50/55lbs – ca. 20kg)

10 rounds
For time

## „ZEUS"

- 30 Wallballs

- 30 Sumo Deadlift High-pull (M=75lbs – ca. 30kg, F=50/55lbs – ca. 20kg)
- 30 Box jump, 20" box
- 30 Push Press (M=75lbs – ca. 30kg, F=50/55lbs – ca. 20kg)
- 30 kcal Row
- 30 Push-ups
- 10 Back Squat Body Weight

3 rounds
For time

## „CAMERON"

- 50 Steps Walking Lunge
- 25 Chest to Bar Pull-ups
- 50 Box Jumps 24"
- 25 Triple Unders
- 50 Back Extensions
- 25 Ring Dips
- 50 Knees to Elbows
- 25 Wallballs "2-fer-1s"
- 50 Sit-ups
- 15 ft (ca. 4,5m) Rope Climb 5 Ascends

For time

## „JORGE"

- 30 GHD Sit-ups
- 15 Squat Clean 155lbs (ca. 70kg)
- 24 GHD Sit-ups
- 12 Squat Clean 155lbs (ca. 70kg)
- 18 GHD Sit-ups
- 9 Squat Clean 155lbs (ca. 70kg)
- 12 GHD Sit-ups

- 6 Squat Clean 155lbs (ca. 70kg)
- 6 GHD Sit-ups
- 3 Squat Clean 155lbs (ca. 70kg)

For time

## „FALKEL"

- 8 Handstand Push-ups
- 8 Box Jump 30" box
- 15 ft (ca. 4,5m) Rope Climb 1 Aufstieg

AMRAP: As Many Rounds As Possible in 20min

## „DOBOGAI"

- 8 Muscle-ups
- 22 yard Farmer carry, 50 pound (ca. 20kg) Dumbbells

7 rounds
For time

## „DG"

- 8 Toes to bar
- 8 Thrusters w/Dumbbells (M=35lbs – ca. 15kg, F=25lbs – ca. 10kg)
- 12 Walking Lunges w/Dumbbells (M=35lbs – ca. 15kg, F=25lbs – ca. 10kg)

AMRAP: As Many Rounds As Possible in 10min

## „TK"

- 8 Strict Pull-ups
- 8 Box Jumps 36"
- 12 Kettlebell Swings (M=2 pood/apx. 72lbs – ca. 30kg, F=50lbs – ca. 20kg)

AMRAP: As Many Rounds As Possible in 20min

## „TK2"

- Body-weight back squats
- Body-weight bench presses
- Strict pull-ups

30-20-10 Repetitions
For time

# BODYWEIGHT

## „100 PULL-UPS"

100 Pull-ups

For time

## „3 TYPES OF PULL-UPS"

- 3 Weighted Pull-ups (45lbs – ca. 20kg)
- 5 Strict Pull-ups
- 7 Kipping Pull-ups

10 rounds
For time

## „TABATA SOMETHING ELSE"

- Pull-ups
- Push-ups
- Sit-ups
- Squats

32 Tabata Intervalls (20s Work - 10s Rest)
Score = sum of all repetitions

## „TABATA THIS"

- Squats
- Row
- Pull-ups
- Sit-ups

- Push-ups

20 Tabata Intervalls (20s Work - 10s Rest)
Score = the fewest number of repetitions of an exercise

## „SBW1"

- 15 Handstand Push-ups
- 1 L-Pull-up
- 13 Handstand Push-ups
- 3 L-Pull-up
- 11 Handstand Push-ups
- 5 L-Pull-up
- 9 Handstand Push-ups
- 7 L-Pull-up
- 7 Handstand Push-ups
- 9 L-Pull-up
- 5 Handstand Push-ups
- 11 L-Pull-up
- 3 Handstand Push-ups
- 13 L-Pull-up
- 1 Handstand Push-ups
- 15 L-Pull-up

For time

## „SBW2"

- 21 L-pull-ups
- 20 One legged squats, alternating legs
- 18 L-pull-ups
- 16 One legged squats, alternating legs
- 15 L-pull-ups
- 12 One legged squats, alternating legs

- 12 L-pull-ups
- 8 One legged squats, alternating legs

For time

## „SBW3"

(100ft = ca. 25m)

- Walking lunge 100 ft.
- 21 Pull-ups
- 21 Sit-ups
- Walking lunge 100 ft.
- 18 Pull-ups
- 18 Sit-ups
- Walking lunge 100 ft.
- 15 Pull-ups
- 15 Sit-ups
- Walking lunge 100 ft.
- 12 Pull-ups
- 12 Sit-ups
- Walking lunge 100 ft.
- 9 Pull-ups
- 9 Sit-ups
- Walking Lunge 100 ft.
- 6 Pull-ups
- 6 Sit-ups

For time

## „SBW4"

- 12 Muscle-ups
- 75 Squats

3 rounds
For time

---

„SBW5"

- 10 Weighted Pull-ups
- 30 Back Extensions

3 rounds
For time

---

„SBW6"

- 30 Glute-Ham Sit-ups
- 25 Back Extensions

5 rounds
For time

---

„SBW7"

- 20 GHD Sit-ups
- 5 Push jerk

5 rounds
For time

---

„SBW7"

- 10 Wall Climbs
- 10 Toes to Bar

- 20 Box Jumps, 24" Box

5 rounds
For time

## „SBW8"

- 5 Handstand Push-ups
- 10 L Pull-ups
- 15 Steps, Walking Lunge

AMRAP: As Many Rounds As Possible in 20min

## „SBW9"

- 15 Pull-ups
- 15 Ring Push-ups
- 15 Back Extensions
- 15 GHD Sit-ups

AMRAP: As Many Rounds As Possible in 20min

## „SBW10"

Death by Pull-ups

1 rep in the first minute, 2 reps in the second minute, 3 reps in the third minute, …
Do until you have to give up

## „SBW11"

Death by Push-ups

1 rep in the first minute, 2 reps in the second minute, 3 reps in the third minute, ...
Do until you have to give up

---

„SBW12"

- Handstand Push-ups 15-13-11-9-7-5-3-1
- L-Pull-ups 1-3-5-7-9-11-13-15

Ascending/Descending
For time

---

„SBW13"

Death by Squats

2 reps in the first minute, 4 reps in the second minute, 6 reps in the third minute, ...
Do until you have to give up

---

„SBW14"

L-Sit 5min

Unimportant how many sets and reps needed
As much reps as possible

---

„SBW15"

100 L-Pull-ups

For time

## „SBW16" – THE 1.000

- Pull-ups
- Push-ups
- Squats
- Crunches

Unimportant how many sets you have to do
Add all repetitions till you have done 1.000 in total

## „SBW17" – THE PLANKS

- Front Plank 1min
- Side Plank (right) 30s
- Side Plank (left) 30s
- Backplank 30s
- Pause 60s

10 rounds

## „SBW18" – LEG CRUSHER

- 25 Squats
- 20 Lunges
- 15 Jump Squats
- 10 Box Jumps
- 6 Pistol Squats (one-leg Squats)

4 rounds
For time

## „SBW19" – STATICS

- 15s L-Sit
- 30s V-Sit
- 60s Plank
- 90s Static Squats (leaning against a wall)

5 rounds


## „SBW20" – THE COUNTDOWN

- Push-up
- Pull-up
- Box Jumps
- Crunches

10-9-8-7-6-5-4-3-2-1 Repetitions
For time

## FREE WEIGHTS

Use a barbell with every exercise, apart from Crunches and Sit-ups

### „BEAR COMPLEX"

Barbell with appr. ¾ Bodyweight, each for 10 reps

- Power Clean
- Front Squat
- Push Press
- Back Squat
- Push Press

5 rounds, rest as needed
For time

### „SFW1"

(ca. 95lbs = ca. 40kg)

- 5 Thruster 95lbs
- 7 Hang Power Cleans 95lbs
- 10 Sumo-Deadlift High-Pull 95lbs

5 rounds
For time

### „SFW2"

95lbs = ca. 40kg

- 10 Power clean 95lbs
- 10 Back Squat 95lbs
- 10 Thruster 95lbs

5 rounds
For time

## „SFW3"

95lbs = ca. 40kg

- 5 Front Squat 95lbs
- 5 Push Press 95lbs
- 5 Sumo-Deadlift High-Pull 95lbs

10 rounds
For time

## „SFW4"

Use ½ Bodyweight

- 10 Front Squat
- 10 Back Squat
- 20 Lunge

7 rounds
For time

## „SFW5"

Use a Dumbbell with appr. ¼ Bodyweight, 8 reps

- Power clean
- Snatch
- Butterfly
- Squat

- Crunch (use a dumbbell too and place your straight arms behind your head holding it)

8 rounds
For time

## „SFW6"

Use Dumbbells with appr. ¼ Bodyweight, 10 reps

- Push Press
- Crunch
- Push Press
- Squat
- Push Press
- Row

3 rounds
For time

## „SFW7"

100 Thruster 95lbs (ca. 40kg)

For time

## „SFW8"

- 10 Front Squat (Barbell ½ Bodyweight)
- 10 Front Squat (Dumbbell ¼ Bodyweight)
- Rest 60s

8 rounds
For time

## „SFW9"

- Benchpress (Dumbbell ¼ Bodyweight)
- Row (Barbell ½ Bodyweight)
- Front Squat (Dumbbell ¼ Bodyweight)

5 rounds
For time

## „SFW10"

250 Power clean (Use any weight)

For time

## „SFW11"

95 lbs = ca. 40kg

- 50Thruster 95lbs
- 150 Hang Power Cleans 95lbs

5 rounds
For time

## „SFW12"

95lbs = ca. 40kg

- 100 Thruster 95lbs
- 100 Front Squats 95 lbs
- 100 Row 95lbs

For time

## „SFW13"

- Front Squat 3min
- Benchpress 3min
- Row 3min
- Snatch 3min

Maximum repetitions

## „SFW14"

250 Hang Power Cleans 95lbs (ca. 40kg)

For time

## „SFW15"

250 Power clean (Use any weight)

For time

## „SFW16"

15min Push Press (Use any weight)

Maximum repetitions

## „SFW17"

Each for one minute, use appr. ¾ Bodyweight, Barbell

- Front Squat
- Front Lunge
- Back Lunge
- Back Squat

Maximum repetitions

## „SFW18"

- 10 Benchpress (Barbell ½ Bodyweight)
- 10 Benchpress (Dumbbell ¼ Bodyweight)
- 10 Benchpress (Barbell ½ Bodyweight)
- 10 Benchpress (Dumbbell ¼ Bodyweight)
- Rest 60s

3 rounds
For time

## „SFW19"

95lbs = ca. 40kg

- Power clean 95lbs
- Deadlift 95lbs

10-9-8-7-6-5-4-3-2-1 Repetitions, Rest as long as you need

## „SFW20"

95lbs = ca. 40kg

- Front Squat 95lbs

- Sumo-Deadlift High-Pull 95lbs

1-2-3-4-5-6-7-8-9-10 Repetitions, Rest as long as you need

## KETTLEBELL

Use a Kettlebell with every exercise, use any weights

### „SK1"

- Front Squat
- Bent Row
- Push-ups

22-16-10 Repetitions
For time

### „SK2"

With 2 Kettlebells

- 10 Thruster
- 20 Snatch
- 30 Alternate Floor Press
- 40 Swing
- 50 Alternate Shoulder Press
- 30 Step-up

For time

### „SK3"

- 3 Snatch (each arm)
- 5 Burpee

AMRAP: As many rounds as possible in 20min

## „SK4"

- 20 Burpee
- 18 Suitcase Deadlift
- 16 Push-ups
- 14 Clean
- 12 Pull-up (Kettlebell between the feet)
- 10 Push Press

2 rounds
For time

## „SK5"

- 3 Back Squat
- 6 Double Kettlebell Swing
- 9 Push-ups

AMRAP: As many rounds as possible in 7min

## „SK6"

- 5 Burpee
- 10 Swing
- 15 Bar dips (Kettlebell between the feet)

AMRAP: As many rounds as possible in 20min

## „SK7"

- 60 Crunches (Kettlebell in hands)
- 50 Suitcase Deadlifts
- 40 Push-ups

- 30 Sumo High Pull
- 20 Burpee
- 10 Pistol Squats (one-leg Squats)

For time

## „SK8"

- 10 Double Jerk
- 8 Snatch (each arm)
- 5 Handstand Push-ups (on Kettelbells)

5 rounds
For time

## „SK9"

- 5 Benchpress
- 7 Double Snatch

5 rounds
For time

## „SK10"

- Snatch 1-2-3-4-5-6 ... -14-15 Repetitions
- Push-ups 15-14-13-12 ... -2-1 Repetitions

For time

## „SK11"

- 6 Snatch
- 12 Box Jumps (Kettlebell in hands)

10 rounds
For time

## „SK12"

- Snatch (alternating right and left)
- Handstand Push-up

21-15-9 Repetitions
For time

## „SK13"

- 8 Single arm Thruster
- 8 Pistols (one-leg Squats)
- 8 Back Lunge

8 rounds
For time

## „SK14"

- 100 Swings
- 100 Goblet Squats
- 100 Press
- 100 Suitcase Deadlift
- 100 Thruster

For time

## „SK15"

- 20 Swing
- 30 Thruster
- 20 Push-ups
- 30 Crunches
- 20 Sumo Deadlift
- 30 Swing

For time

## „SK16"

- 20 Swing
- 15 Push-up
- 10 Sumo Deadlift
- 5 Pistol (one-leg Squat)

5 rounds
For time

## „SK17"

- 10 Snatch (alternating right and left)
- 10 Push-ups

AMRAP: As many rounds as possible in 10min

## „SK18"

Clean and Jerk

1-2-3-2-3-4-3-4-5-4-5-6-5-6-7-6-7-8 Repetitions
For time

## „SK19"

250 Swing

For time

## „SK20"

- 30 Front Squat
- 30 Push-ups
- 10 Snatch
- 10 Pull-ups (Kettlebell between the feet)

3 rounds
For time

# MIXED

## „NASTY GIRL"

- 50 Squats
- 7 Muscle-ups
- 10 Hang Power Cleans 135lbs (ca. 65kg)

3 rounds
For time

## „THE 45'S"

- 45 Double Unders
- 45 Squat Clean 135lbs (ca. 60kg)
- 45 Ring Dips
- 45 Double Unders

For time

## „THE CHIEF"

Maximum rounds in 3min:

- 3 Power Cleans 135lbs (ca. 60kg)
- 6 Push-ups
- 9 Squat

5 rounds with 1min rest between the rounds
Score = Sum of all repetitions

## „THE NAMELESS WORKOUTS"

- 75 Push-ups
- 50 Sumo-Deadlift High-Pull 95lbs (ca. 40kg)
- 50 Ring Dips
- 30 Weighted Pull-ups 45lb (ca. 20kg)
- 25 Handstand Push-ups

For time

## „SM1"

- 10 GHD Sit-ups
- 10 Hip & Back Extensions
- 30 Thrusters 95lbs (ca. 40kg)
- 50 Pull-ups
- 30 GHD Sit-ups
- 30 Hip & Back Extensions
- 20 Thrusters 95lbs (ca. 40kg)
- 35 Pull-ups
- 50 GHD Sit-ups
- 50 Hip & Back Extensions
- 10 Thrusters 95lbs (ca. 40kg)
- 20 Pull-ups

For time

## „SM2"

(ca. 155lbs = ca. 70kg)

- 15 Power Clean 155lbs
- 30 Ring Dips
- 12 Power Clean 155lbs
- 24 Ring Dips
- 9 Power Clean 155lbs
- 18 Ring Dips

- 6 Power Clean 155lbs
- 12 Ring Dips
- 3 Power Clean 155lbs
- 6 Ring Dips

For time

## „SM3"

- 50 box Jumps 20" Box
- Rope climb 5 Ascends
- 50 Kettlebell Swing 1.5 pood (apx 55lbs – ca. 25kg)
- 50 Sit-ups
- 50 Hang power clean 40lb (ca. 20kg) Dumbbell
- 800m Run
- 50 Back extensions

For time

## „SM4"

- 6 Muscle-ups
- 30 Wallball 20lbs (ca. 8kg)
- 12 Handstand Push-ups
- 15 Power clean 135lbs (ca. 65kg)

3 rounds
For time

## „SM5"

- 10 Deadlift 275lbs (ca. 130kg)
- 50 Double unders

3 rounds
For time

## „SM6"

- 3 Deadlifts
- Handstand Push-ups, max. reps

5 rounds
For time and maximum repetitions

## „SM7"

- 10 Sumo-Deadlift High-Pulls 95lbs (ca. 40kg)
- 10 Ring Dips

7 rounds
For time

## „SM8"

- 3 Front Squat 185lbs (ca. 85kg)
- 7 L-Pull-ups

7 rounds
For time

## „SM9"

- 10 Thrusters 65lbs (ca. 30kg)
- 10 Pull-ups

AMRAP: As Many Rounds As Possible in 20min

## „SM10"

- 5 Chest to bar Pull-ups
- 10 Ring Dips
- 15 Overhead Squat 95lbs (ca. 45kg)

AMRAP: As Many Rounds As Possible in 20min

## „SM11" – CHEST

- 10 Benchpress (Bodyweight)
- 10 Butterfly (Dumbbell – ¼ Bodyweight)
- 20 Push-ups
- 10 Pull-over (Barbell –1/3 Bodyweight)

3 rounds
For time

## „SM12" – BACK

- 10 Deadlift (Bodyweight)
- 10 Row (Barbell – 2/3 Bodyweight)
- 10 Pull-ups
- 20 Butterfly reverse (Dumbbell – ¼ Bodyweight)

3 rounds
For time

## „SM13" – LEGS

- 15 Squats (Barbell - ¾ Bodyweight)
- 20 Box Jumps
- 15 Deadlifts (Barbell – ¾ Bodyweight)
- 6 Pistol Squats (one-leg Squats)

3 rounds
For time

## „SM14" – FULL BODY ROUTINE

- Deadlift (Bodyweight)
- Pull-ups
- Push-ups
- Crunches
- Squats (Bodyweight)
- 60s Rest

3 rounds
Maximum repetitions

## „SM15" – ONLY 2

- 25 Push-ups
- 25 Deadlift (3/4 Bodyweight)

5 rounds
For time

## „SM16" – DUMBBELL/BARBELL

- 20 Overhead Squats (Barbell – ½ Bodyweight)
- 20 Benchpress (Barbell – ½ Bodyweight)
- 20 Overhead Squats (Dumbbell – ¼ Bodyweight)

- 20 Benchpress (Dumbbell – ¼ Bodyweight)

3 rounds
For time

## „SM17"

- 100 Snatch (1/2 Bodyweight)
- 100 Deadlifts (1/2 Bodyweight)
- 100 Push-ups

For time

## „SM18" 5X5X5

- 5 Squats (Bodyweight)
- 5 Push-ups
- 5 Deadlifts (Bodyweight)
- 5 Pull-ups
- 5 Crunches

5 rounds
For time

## „SM19"

- 100 Power clean (½ Bodyweight)
- 100 Pull-ups

For time

## „SM20" – GIVE UP

- 500 Snatch (½ Bodyweight)
- 500 Benchpress (½ Bodyweight)
- 500 Box Jumps

Anyhow
For time

## ENDURANCE ONLY

The WOD'S in this category focus primarily on endurance and speed.

### RUN

#### „ER1" – PICK A DISTANCE

Run: 1mile, 2miles, 5km, 8km, 10km, 15km, 13,1miles

For time (each)

#### „ER2" – PICK A TIME

Run: 20min, 30min, 40min, 60min, 90min

Maximum distance (each)

#### „ER3"

- Run: 5min max. Distance
- Walking: 3min Recovery

4 rounds

#### „ER4"

- Run: 5k
- Walking: 10min Recovery

3 rounds

„ER5"

- 1200m uphill Sprint
- 1min Rest
- 1200m downhill Run
- 1min Rest

3 rounds
For time

„ER6"

10x 100m Sprint with 2min rest

„ER7"

8x 200m Sprint with 2min rest

„ER8"

4x 400m Sprint with 5min rest

„ER9"

- 80s Sprint
- 40s Rest

8 rounds

## „ER10"

- Run: 1min
- Walking: 1min Recovery
- Run: 2min
- Walking: 2min Recovery
- Run: 3min
- Walking: 3min Recovery

3 rounds
Maximum distance

## „ER11"

- 100m Sprint
- Rest, as long as it took to sprint 100m
- 200m Sprint
- Rest, as long as it took to sprint 200m
- 300m Sprint
- Rest, as long as it took to sprint 300m

3 rounds
For time

## „ER12"

- 10s Sprint
- 5s Rest

8 rounds
Maximum distance

## „ER13"

- 1min Sprint
- 1min Rest

10 rounds
Maximum distance

## „ER14"

- 10s Sprint
- 20s Rest

16 rounds
Maximum distance

## „ER15" – TABATA SPRINT

- 20s Sprint
- 10s Rest

8 rounds
Maximum distance

## „ER16"

- 3min Run
- 1min Rest
- 3min Run
- 3min Rest

2 rounds
Maximum distance

„ER17"

- 400m Run
- 2min Rest

6 rounds
For time


„ER18"

- 1600m Run
- 4min Rest
- 1200m Run
- 3min Rest
- 800m Run
- 2min Rest
- 400m Run
- 1min Rest
- 200m Run

For time


„ER19"

- 50m Run
- 10s Rest
- 100m Run
- 20s Rest
- 200m Run
- 30s Rest
- 400m Run
- 45s Rest
- 800m Run
- 60s Rest

2 rounds
For time

## „ER20"

- Downhill Sprint
- 1min Rest
- Uphill Sprint
- 1min Rest

5 rounds
For time

# SWIM

## „ES1" - PICK A DISTANCE

Swim: 250m, 500m, 1k, 1,5k, 2k

For time (each)

## „ES2" – PICK A TIME

Swim: 10min, 20min, 30min, 45min, 60min, 90min

Maximum distance (each)

## „ES3"

- Freestyle: 25m
- Recovery: 30s

10 rounds
For time

## „ES4"

- Freestyle: 50m
- Backstroke: 50m
- Recovery: 60s

5 rounds
For time

## „ES5"

- Backstroke: 250m
- Recovery: 60s

4 rounds
For time

## „ES6"

- Breaststroke: 25m
- Freestyle: 25m
- Backstroke: 25m
- Butterfly: 25m

10 rounds
For time

## „ES7"

- Freestyle 500m
- Recovery: 60s
- Breaststroke: 500m
- Recovery: 60s

3 rounds
For time

## „ES8"

- 25m Sprint – Freestyle
- 60s Recovery

10 rounds
For time

## „ES9"

- Backstroke: 5min
- 25m Sprint – Freestyle
- Recovery: 60s
- Breaststroke: 5min
- 25 Sprint – Freestyle
- Recovery: 60s
- Butterfly: 5min
- 25m Sprint - Freestyle

Maximum distance

## „ES10"

- 25m Freestyle
- 25m Sprint – Freestyle

10 rounds
For time

## „ES11"

- 250m Freestyle
- 25m Sprint – Butterfly
- 250m Freestyle
- 25m Sprint – Backstroke
- 250m Freestyle
- 25m Sprint – Breaststroke

For time

## „ES12"

- 500m Butterfly

Rest as long as you need
For time

## „ES13"

- 2 Strokes Breaststroke
- 4 Strokes Freestyle
- for 50m
- 4 Strokes Freestyle
- 4 Strokes Backstroke
- for 50m

10 rounds
For time

## „ES14"

1000m Swim, no Freestyle

For time

## „ES15"

10.000m Swim

Anyhow

## „ES16"

- 500m Swim (Use any technique)
- 2min Rest

2 rounds
For time

## „ES17"

Freestyle

- 25m Swim
- 10s Rest
- 50m Swim
- 30s Rest
- 100m Swim
- 60s Rest
- 250m Swim
- 2min Rest

3 rounds
For time

## „ES18"

- 200m Freestyle
- 200m Backstroke
- 200m Breaststroke
- 100m Butterfly
- 300m Freestyle

Rest as long as you need
For time

## „ES19"

- 50m Breaststroke
- 60s Rest
- 50m Breaststroke
- 40s Rest
- 50m Breaststroke
- 20s Rest
- 50m Breaststroke
- 10s Rest

3 rounds
For time

## „ES20"

Swim - Freestyle

10-9-8-7-6-5-4-3-2-1 Lanes

60s Rest between the sets
For time

## „ES21"

Swim – Freestyle

1-2-3-4-5-6-7-8-9-10 Lanes

60s Rest between the sets
For time

# ROW

Sprint exercises within the Row WOD'S mean row-sprints.

## „ERW1"

- Row 1min
- Rest 1min
- Row 1min
- Rest 50s
- Row 1min
- Rest 40s
- Row 1min
- Rest 30s
- Row 1min
- Rest 20s
- Row 1min
- Rest 10s

2 rounds
Maximum distance

## „ERW2"

- 60s Row
- 60s Rest

10 rounds
Maximum distance

## „ERW3"

- 90s Row
- 90s Rest

6 rounds

Maximum distance

## „ERW4"

- 100m Row
- 100m Sprint
- 80m Row
- 100m Sprint
- 60m Row
- 100m Sprint
- 40m Row
- 100m Sprint
- 20m Row
- 100m Sprint

For time

## „ERW5" – PICK A DISTANCE

Row – 500m, 1000m, 1500m, 2000m, 2500m

For time (each)

## „ERW6" – PICK A TIME

Row – 5min, 10min, 15min, 25min, 45min, 60min, 90min

Maximum distance (each)

## „ERW7"

- 250m Row
- 45s Rest

8 rounds
For time

## „ERW8"

Ratio (Row:Rest)

- 1:1
- 2:1
- 3:1
- 4:1
- 1:1

5 rounds

## „ERW9"

- 45m Row
- 10m Rest

20 rounds
For time

## „ERW10"

- 2min Row
- 1min Rest

4 rounds
Maximum distance

## „ERW11"

- 30s Row
- 2min Rest

10 rounds
Maximum distance

## „ERW12"

- 250m Row
- Rest (same amount of time as you needed for the 250m)

5 rounds
For time

## „ERW13"

- 3000m Row
- 2min Rest

2 rounds
For time

## „ERW14"

2000m Row

Do as many sprints of 50m as you can within the 2000m rowing

„ERW15"

- 250m Row
- 1min Rest
- 500m Row
- 1min Rest
- 750m Row
- 1min Rest

3 rounds
For time


„ERW16"

- 1000m Row
- 1min Rest

3 rounds
For time


„ERW17"

- 100m Row
- 25m Sprint
- 100m Row
- 50m Sprint

8 rounds
For time


„ERW18"

- 500m Row

- 3min Rest

4 rounds
For time

## „ERW19"

- 100m Row
- 30s Rest
- 100m Row
- 20s Rest
- 100m Row
- 10s Rest

8 rounds
For time

## „ERW20"

- 500m Row
- 50m Sprint

5 rounds
For time

## BIKING

Sprint exercises within the Biking category mean bike-sprints.

### „EB1" – PICK A DISTANCE

Bike – 5km, 10km, 20km, 30km, 45km, 75km, 100km, 5miles, 10miles, 20miles, 50miles

For time (each)

### „EB2" – PICK A TIME

Bike – 15min, 30min, 45min, 60min, 9min, 120min

Maximum distance (each)

### „EB3"

- 5min Bike
- 3min Rest

5 rounds
Maximum distance

### „EB4"

- 15km
- 2min Rest

4 rounds
For time

## „EB5"

- 1km Uphill
- 1km Downhill

10 rounds
For time

## „EB6"

- 500m Bike
- 500m Sprint

8 rounds
For time

## „EB7"

- 1000m Sprint
- 2min Rest

8 rounds
For time

## „EB8"

- 2500m Sprint
- 500m Bike

4 rounds
For time

„EB9"

- 1min Sprint
- 4min Bike

10 rounds
Maximum distance

„EB10"

- 1000m Bike
- 60s Rest
- 1000m Bike
- 45s Rest
- 1000m Bike
- 30s Rest
- 1000m Bike
- 15s Rest

2 rounds
For time

„EB11"

10.000m Bike with as many sprints as possible

Increase the number of sprints with every WOD

„EB12"

- 20s Sprint
- 10s Bike

8 rounds
Maximum distance

## „EB13"

- 1min Sprint
- 1min Bike

12 rounds
Maximum distance

## „EB14"

- 10s Sprint
- 20s Bike

12 rounds
Maximum distance

## „EB15"

- 5000m Bike
- 1min Rest
- 4000m Bike
- 1min Rest
- 2000m Bike
- 1min Rest
- 1000m Bike
- 1min Rest
- 500m Sprint

For time

„EB16"

- 400m Sprint
- 100m Rest

10 rounds
For time


„EB17"

- 200m Sprint
- 200m Bike
- 400m Sprint
- 400m Bike
- 800m Sprint
- 800m Bike
- 1600m Sprint
- 1600m Bike

For time


„EB18"

- 200m Sprint
- 200m Bike
- 200m Sprint
- 100m Bike
- 200m Sprint
- 50m Bike

8 rounds
For time

## „EB19"

- 2min Sprint
- 2min Bike
- 2min Sprint
- 1min Bike
- 2min Sprint
- 30s Bike

8 rounds
For time

## „EB20" – PICK A DISTANCE UPHILL

Uphill Bike – 500m, 1km, 2km, 5km, 10km

For time (each)

# INLINER

Sprint exercises within the Inliner WOD'S mean skating-sprints

## „EI1" PICK A DISTANCE

Skate – 1km, 2km, 5km, 10km, 25km

For time (each)

## „EI2" PICK A TIME

Skate – 5min, 15min, 25min, 45min, 60min, 90min

For distance (each)

## „EI3"

- 5min Skate
- 1min Rest

5 rounds
Maximum distance

## „EI4"

- 2km Skate
- 3min Rest

3 rounds
For time

## „E15"

- 200m Uphill
- 200m Downhill

10 rounds
For time

## „E16"

10x 100m Sprints with 60s Rest

For time

## „E17"

10x 200m Sprints with 2min Rest

For time

## „E18"

- 400m Skate
- 400m Sprint

8 rounds
For time

## „E19"

- 1min Sprint
- 30s Skate

12 rounds
Maximum distance

## „EI10"

- 1min Sprint
- 2min Skate
- 2min Sprint
- 2min Skate
- 3min Sprint
- 2min Skate

3 rounds
Maximum distance

## „EI11"

- 100m Sprint
- 100m Rollout
- 200m Sprint
- 100m Rollout
- 400m Sprint
- 100m Rollout

5 rounds
For time

## „EI12"

- 10s Sprint
- 20s Rollout

12 rounds
Maximum distance

## „EI13"

- 20s Sprint
- 10s Rollout

8 rounds
Maximum distance

## „EI14"

- 60s Sprint
- 60s Skate
- 60s Rollout

10 rounds
Maximum distance

## „EI15"

- 3min Skate
- 1min Rollout
- 5min Skate
- 1min Rollout
- 1min Sprint
- 1min Rollout

8 rounds
Maximum distance

„EI16"

- 2km Skate
- 500m Sprint
- 1min Rollout

4 rounds
For time

„EI17"

- 2500m Skate
- 1min Rollout
- 2000m Skate
- 1min Rollout
- 1500m Skate
- 1min Rollout
- 1000m Skate
- 1min Rollout
- 500m Skate
- 1min Rollout
- 250m Sprint

For time

„EI18"

- 10s Sprint
- 30s Rollout
- 20s Sprint
- 30s Rollout
- 30s Sprint
- 30s Rollout

8 rounds
Maximum distance

## „EI19"

5000m Skate with as many sprints of 50m as possible

For time

## „EI20"

- 1000m Skate
- 1000m Skate (in ¾ of the time you needed for the first Intervall)
- 1000m Skate (in ½ of the time you needed for the first Intervall)
- 1000m as fast as possible

For time

## ENDURANCE-EXERCISES

### „EE1" – BURPEE MILE

1mile Burpees

For time

### „EE2" – DEATH BY BURPEES

- One Burpee in the first minute
- Two Burpees in the second minute
- Three Burpees in the third minute
- ...

Do until you have to stop

### „EE3"

- 10 Burpees
- 30s Rest

8 rounds
For time

### „EE4"

250 Burpees

For time

## „EE5" DEATH BY JUMPING JAKCS

- 2 Jumping Jacks in the first minute
- 4 Jumping Jacks in the second minute
- 6 Jumping Jacks in the third minute
- ...

Do until you have to stop

## „EE6"

1000 Jumping Jacks

For time

## „EE7"

- 20s Jumping Jacks
- 10s Rest

10 rounds
As many reps as possible

## „EE8" – DEATH BY HIGH KNEES

- 5 High knees in the first minute
- 10 High knees in the second minute
- 15 High knees in the third minute
- ...

Do until you have to stop

## „EE9"

2500 High knees

For time

## „EE10"

- 20s High knees
- 10s Rest

12 rounds
As many reps as possible

## „EE11"

- 10 Burpees
- 25 Jumping Jacks
- 1min Rest

4 rounds
For time

## „EE12"

- 100 Burpees
- 250 Jumping Jacks

For time

## „EE13"

- 10 Burpees
- 50 High knees
- 90s Rest

5 rounds
For time

„EE14"

- 100 Burpees
- 500 High knees

For time

„EE15"

- 25 Jumping Jacks
- 50 High knees
- 30s Rest

3 rounds
For time

„EE16"

- 500 Jumping Jacks
- 1000 High knees

For time

„EE17"

- 5 Burpees
- 10 Jumping Jacks
- 20 High knees
- 1min Rest

4 rounds
For time

## „EE18"

- 20s Burpees
- 10s Rest
- 20s Jumping Jacks
- 10s Rest
- 20s High knees
- 10s Rest

6 rounds
Maximum repetitions

## „EE19"

1 Burpee, 2 Jumping Jacks, 4 High knees

10min in total, do as many reps as possible

## „EE20"

- 100 Burpees
- 250 Jumping Jacks
- 500 High knees

For time

# MIXED-ENDURANCE

## „EM1"

- 500m Row
- 21 Burpees
- 400m Run

3 rounds
For time


## „EM2" – FILTHY FIFTEEN MILES

- 400m Run
- 10 Burpees

60 rounds
For time


## „EM3"

- 50 Jumping Jacks
- Swim: 50m Freestyle

10 rounds
For time


## „EM4"

- 10 Burpees
- Swim: 50m Breaststroke
- 25 Jumping Jacks
- Swim: 50m Freestyle

6 rounds
For time

## „EM5"

- Swim: 25m Freestyle
- 50 High knees
- Swim: 25m Breaststroke
- 50 Jumping Jacks

For time

## „EM6"

- 2500m Row
- 2500m Run

For time

## „EM7"

- 1000m Swim
- 5000m Run

For time

## „EM8"

- 500m Swim
- 5000m Bike
- 2000m Run

For time

## „EM9"

- 2000m Inline
- 1000m Run
- 100 Burpees

For time

## „EM10"

- 10.000m Bike
- 5000m Run

For time

## „EM11"

- 500 High knees
- 5000m Run
- 50 Burpees
- 50m Sprint

For time

## „EM12"

- 50m Sprint
- 5 Burpees
- 1min Rest

10 rounds
For time

## „EM13"

- 25 Jumping Jacks
- 100m Sprint
- 5 Burpees
- 100m Sprint
- 2min Rest

3 rounds
For time

## „EM14"

- 10m Uphill Burpee
- 40m Uphill Sprint
- 10m Uphill Burpee
- 40m Uphill Sprint
- 100m Downhill Run

4 rounds
For time

## „EM15"

- 500m Bike Sprint
- 100m Run Sprint
- 1min Rest
- 100m Run Sprint back
- 500m Bike Sprint back
- 1min Rest

5 rounds
For time

## „EM16"

- 20 High knees
- 400m Run
- 10 Burpees
- 400m Run
- 15 Jumping Jacks
- 400m Run

For time

## „EM17"

- 20s Run
- 10s Rest
- 20s Burpee
- 10s Rest
- 20s Jumping Jack
- 10s Rest
- 20s High knees
- 10s Rest

2 rounds
Maximum repetitions or distance

## „EM18"

- 20s Bike Sprint
- 10s Rest
- 20s Run Sprint

- 10s Rest
- 20s Run Sprint back
- 10s Rest

4 rounds
Maximum effort

## „EM19" – TRIATHLON (OLYMPIC)

- 800m Swim
- 30.000m Bike
- 10.000m Run

For time

## „EM20" – DEATH BY ENDURANCE

Death by Prinzip:

- One rep each in the first minute
- Two rep each in the second minute
- Three rep each in the third minute
- …

Exercises:

- Jumping Jack
- Burpee
- High knees
- 10m Run Sprint

Do every exercise as long as you can do the necessary reps in the specific minute. The WOD is done when you can't do the necessary reps for every exercise in the specific minute.

## STRENGHT/ENDURANCE COMBINED

### BENCHMARK

#### „HELEN"

- 400m Run
- 21 Kettlebell Swing 1.5 pood (apx 55lbs – ca. 20kg)
- 12 Pull-ups

3 rounds
For time

#### „JACKIE"

- 1000m Row
- 50 Thruster 45lbs (ca. 18kg)
- 30 Pull-ups

For time

#### „NANCY"

- 400m Run
- 15 Overhead Squat 95lbs (ca. 40kg)

5 rounds
For time

#### „EVA"

- 800m Run
- 30 Kettlebell Swing 2 pood (apx 72lbs – ca. 30kg)

- 30 Pull-ups

5 rounds
For time

## „KELLY"

- 400m Run
- 30 Box Jump (24" box)
- 30 Wallball 20lbs (ca. 8kg)

5 rounds
For time

## „NICOLE"

- 400m Run
- Max. rep Pull-ups

AMRAP: As Many Rounds As Possible in 20min

# HERO

## „MICHAEL"

- 800m Run
- 50 Back Extensions
- 50 Sit-ups

3 rounds
For time

## MURPH (AKA „BODY ARMOUR")

- 1 mile Run
- 100 Pull-ups
- 200 Push-ups
- 300 Squats
- 1 mile Run

For time

## „DANIEL"

- 50 Pull-ups
- 400m Run
- 21 Thrusters 95lbs (ca. 40kg)
- 800m Run
- 21 Thrusters 95lbs (ca. 40kg)
- 400m Run
- 50 Pull-ups

For time

## „BADGER"

- 30 Squat Cleans 95lbs (ca. 40kg)
- 30 Pull-ups
- 800m Run

3 rounds
For time

## „GRIFF"

- 800m Run
- 400m Run backwards
- 800m Run
- 400m Run backwards

For time

## „RYAN"

- 7 Muscle-ups
- 21 Burpees

5 rounds
For time

## „MR JOSHUA"

- 400m Run
- 30 Glute-Ham Sit-Ups
- 15 Deadlift 250lbs (ca. 115kg)

5 rounds
For time

### „JERRY"

- 1 mile Run
- 2000m Row
- 1 mile Run

For time

### „NUTTS"

- 10 Handstand Push-ups
- 15 Deadlift 250lbs (ca. 115kg)
- 25 Box Jumps, 30" Box
- 50 Pull-ups
- 100 Wallball 20lbs
- 200 Double Unders
- 400m Run with a 45lb (ca. 20kg) plate

For time

### „THE SEVEN"

- 7 Handstand Push-ups
- 7 Thruster 135lbs (ca. 60kg)
- 7 Knees to elbows
- 7 Deadlift 245lbs (ca. 115kg)
- 7 Burpees
- 7 Kettlebell Swings 2 pood (apx 72lbs – ca. 30kg)
- 7 Pull-ups

7 rounds
For time

## „RJ"

(15ft = 4,5m)

- 800m Run
- 15 ft Rope Climb 5 Ascends
- 50 Push-ups

3 rounds
For time


## „LUCE"

Wearing a 20lbs (ca. 10kg) vest:

- Run 1K
- 10 Muscle-ups
- 100 Squats

3 rounds
For time


## „SEVERIN"

- 50 Strict Pull-ups
- 100 Plyo Push-ups (Hands are both in the air for a short amout of time after the pull motion)
- Run 5K

Use a weight vest if possible
For time


## „HELTON"

- 800m Run
- 30 Squat Clean 50lb (ca. 20kg) Dumbbells
- 30 Burpees

3 rounds
For time

## „FORREST"

- 20 L-Pull-ups
- 30 Toes to bar
- 40 Burpees
- 800m Run

3 rounds
For time

## „BULGER"

- 150m Run
- 7 Chest to Bar pull-ups
- 7 Front Squat 135lbs (ca. 60kg)
- 7 Handstand Push-ups

10 rounds
For time

## BRENTON

- Bear Crawl 100ft
- Standing Broad-jump 100ft - ca. 30m (3 Burpees after 5 broadjumps)

Use a weight vest if possible
5 rounds
For time

## „COLLIN"

- Carry 50 pound (ca. 20kg) sandbag 400m
- 12 Push Press 115lbs (ca. 50kg)
- 12 Box jumps 24" Box
- 12 Sumo Deadlift High-pull 95lbs (ca. 40kg)

6 rounds
For time

## „WHITTEN"

- 22 Kettlebell Swings 2 pood (apx 72lbs – ca. 30kg)
- 22 Box jump 24" Box
- 400m Run
- 22 Burpees
- 22 Wallball shots 20lbs (ca. 8kg)

5 rounds
For time

## „BULL"

- 200 Double unders
- 50 Overhead Squat 135lbs (ca. 60kg)
- 50 Pull-ups
- 1 mile Run

2 rounds
For time

## „JOHN RANKEL"

- 6 Deadlift 225lbs (ca. 100kg)
- 7 Burpee Pull-ups
- 10 Kettlebell Swings 2 pood (apx 72lbs – ca. 30kg)

AMRAP: As Many Rounds As Possible in 20min

## „HOLBROOK"

- 5 Thrusters 115lbs (ca. 50kg)
- 10 Pull-ups
- 100m Sprint
- 1min Rest

10 rounds
For time

## „MCCLUSKEY"

- 9 Muscle-ups
- 15 Burpee Pull-ups
- 21 Pull-ups
- 800m Run

3 rounds
For time

## „ABBATE"

- 1 mile Run
- 21 Clean and Jerk 155lbs (ca. 70kg)

- 800m Run
- 21 Clean and Jerk 155lbs (ca. 70kg)
- 1 mile Run

For time

## „MOORE"

- 15 ft (ca. 4,5m) Rope Climb, 1 Ascend
- 400m Run
- Max rep Handstand Push-ups

AMRAP: As Many Rounds As Possible in 20min

## „MOON"

- 10 Right arm Hang Split Snatch 40lb (ca. 15kg) Dumbbell
- 15 ft (ca. 4,5m) Rope Climb 1 Ascend
- 10 Left arm Hang Split Snatch 40lb (ca. 15kg) Dumbbell
- 15 ft (ca. 4,5m) Rope Climb 1 Ascend

7 rounds
For time

## „SMALL"

- 1000m Row
- 50 Burpees
- 50 Box jumps 24" box
- 800m Run

3 rounds
For time

## „MANION"

- 400m Run
- 29 Back Squat (M=135lbs – ca. 60kg, F=95lbs – ca. 40kg)

7 rounds
For time

## „BRADLEY"

- 100m Sprint
- 10 Pull-ups
- 100m Sprint
- 10 Burpees
- 30s Rest

10 rounds
For time

## „WHITE"

- 15 ft (ca. 4,5m) Rope Climb 3 Ascends
- 10 Toes to bar
- 21 Walking lunge steps with 45lb plate (ca. 20kg) Overhead
- Run 400m

5 rounds
For time

## „SANTORA"

- 1min of Squat Cleans 155lbs (ca. 70kg)
- 1min of 20' Shuttle Sprints (20' forward + 20' backwards = 1 rep; 20ft = ca. 10m)
- 1min of Deadlifts 245lbs (ca. 110kg)
- 1min of Burpees
- 1min of Jerks 155lbs (ca. 70kg)
- 1min Rest

3 rounds
For time


## „WOOD"

- 400m Run
- 10 Burpee Box Jumps 24" box
- 10 Sumo-Deadlift High-pull (M=95lbs – ca. 40kg, F=65lbs – ca. 30kg)
- 10 Thruster (M=95lbs – ca. 40kg, F=65lbs – ca. 30kg)
- 1min Rest

5 rounds
For time


## „WAKO"

- 2 mile Run
- 2min Rest
- 20 Squat Clean (M=135lbs – ca. 60kg, F=95lbs – ca. 40kg)
- 20 Box Jump 24"
- 20 Walking Lunge steps with 45lb plate (ca. 20kg) Überkopf
- 20 Box Jump 24"
- 20 Squat Clean (M=135lbs – ca. 60kg, F=95lbs – ca. 40kg)
- 2min Rest
- 2 mile Run

Use a weight vest if possible
For time

## „DAE HAN"

- 800m Run with a 45 pound (ca. 20kg) Barbell
- 15 ft (ca. 4,5m) Rope Climb 3 Ascends
- 12 Thruster (M=135lbs – ca. 60kg, F=95lbs – ca. 40kg)

3 rounds
For time

## „RAHOI"

- 12 Box Jumps 24"
- 6 Thrusters (M=95lbs – ca. 40kg. F=65lbs – ca. 30kg)
- 6 Bar-facing Burpees

AMRAP: As Many Rounds As Possible in 20min

## „KLEPTO"

- 27 Box Jumps 24"
- 20 Burpees
- 11 Squat Cleans 145lbs (ca. 70kg)

4 rounds
For time

## „JAG 28"

- 800m Run
- 28 Kettlebell Swings 2 pood (apx 72lbs – 30kg)
- 28 Strict Pull-ups
- 28 Kettlebell Clean and Jerk 2 pood each
- 28 Strict Pull-ups
- 800m Run

For time

## „STRANGE"

- 600m Run
- 11 Weighted Pull-up 1.5 pood (apx. 55lbs – 20kg)
- 11 Steps Walking Lunge carrying 1.5 pood Kettlebells
- 11 Thruster 1.5 pood Kettlebell

8 rounds
For time

## „TUMILSON"

- 200m Run
- 11 Burpee Deadlifts 60lb (ca. 25kg) Dumbbells

8 rounds
For time

## „JARED"

- 800m Run
- 40 Pull-ups
- 70 Push-ups

4 rounds
For time

## „TULLY"

- 200m Swim
- 23 Squat Cleans 40lbs (ca. 15kg) Dumbbells

4 rounds
For time

## „GLEN"

- 30 Clean and Jerk (M=135lbs – ca. 60kg, F=95lbs – ca. 40kg)
- 1 mile Run
- 15 ft (ca. 4,5m) Rope Climb 10 Ascends
- 1 mile Run
- 100 Burpees

For time

## „RALPH"

- 8 Deadlift 250lbs (ca. 120kg)
- 16 Burpees
- 15 ft (ca. 4,5m) Rope Climb 3 Ascends
- 600m Run

4 rounds
For time

## „CLOVIS"

- 10 mile Run
- 150 Burpee Pull-ups

For time

## „WESTON"

- 1000m Row
- 200m Farmer carry 45lb (ca. 20kg) Dumbbells
- 50m Right arm Waiter Walk 45lbs (ca. 20kg) Dumbbell
- 50m Left arm Waiter Walk 45lbs (ca. 20kg) Dumbbell

5 rounds
For time

## „LOREDO"

- 24 Squats
- 24 Push-ups
- 24 Steps Walking Lunge
- 400m Run

6 rounds
For time

## „HORTMAN"

- 800m Run
- 80 Squats
- 8 Muscle-ups

AMRAP: As Many Rounds As Possible in 45min

## „HAMILTON"

- 1000m Row
- 50 Push-ups
- 1000m Run
- 50 Pull-ups

3 rounds
For time

## „BARRAZA"

- 200m Run
- 9 Deadlift 275lbs (ca. 130kg)
- 6 Burpee Bar Muscle-ups

AMRAP: As Many Rounds As Possible in 18min

## „BREHM"

- 15 ft (4,5m) Rope Climb 10 Ascends
- 20 Back Squat 225lbs (ca. 100kg)
- 30 Handstand Push-ups
- Row 40kcal

For time

## „OMAR"

- 10 Thrusters (M=95lbs – ca. 45kg, F=65lbs – ca. 30kg)
- 15 Bar-facing burpees
- 20 Thrusters (M=95lbs - ca. 45kg, F=65lbs – ca. 30kg)
- 25 Bar-facing burpees
- 30 Thrusters (M=95lbs – ca. 45kg, F=65lbs – ca. 30kg)
- 35 Bar-facing burpees

For time

## „GALLANT"

- 1 mile Run with a 20 pound (ca. 8kg) medicine ball
- 60 Burpee pull-ups
- 800m Run with a 20 pound (ca. 8kg) medicine ball
- 30 Burpee pull-ups
- 400m Run with a 20 pound (ca. 8kg) medicine ball
- 15 Burpee pull-ups

For time

## „SMYKOWSKI"

- 6K Run
- 60 Burpee Pull-ups

Use a weight vest if possible
For time

## „DONNY"

- Deadlift 225lbs (ca. 100kg)
- Burpees

21-15-9-9-15-21 Repetitions
For time

## „RONEY"

- 200m Run
- 11 Thruster (M=135lbs – ca. 60kg, F=95lbs – ca. 40kg)
- 200m Run
- 11 Push Press (M=135lbs –ca. 60kg, F=95lbs – ca. 40kg)
- 200m Run
- 11 Bench Press (M=135lbs – ca. 60kg, F=95lbs – ca. 40kg)

4 rounds
For time

## „DON"

- 66 Deadlifts (M=110lbs – ca. 50kg, F=75lbs – ca. 35kg)
- 66 Box jump (M=24", F=18/20")
- 66 Kettlebell Swings (M=1.5 pood, F=1.0 pood)
- 66 Knees to Elbows
- 66 Sit-ups
- 66 Pull-ups
- 66 Thrusters (M=55lbs - ca. 20kg, F=35/40lbs – ca. 15kg)
- 66 Wallballs
- 66 Burpees
- 66 Double Unders

For time

## „DRAGON"

- 5k Run

- 4min to find 4 rep max. Deadlift
- 5k Run
- 4min to find 4 rep max. Push jerk

For time and maximum weight

## „WALSH"

- 22 Burpee Pull-ups
- 22 Back Squat (M=185lbs – ca. 85kg,F=125/130lbs – ca. 60kg)
- 200m Run with a 45lb (ca. 20kg) plate Overhead

4 rounds
For time

## „LEE"

- 400m Run
- 1 Deadlift 345lbs (160kg)
- 3 Squat Clean 185lbs (ca. 85kg)
- 5 Push Jerk 185lbs (ca. 85kg)
- 3 Muscle-ups
- 15 ft (ca. 4,5m) Rope climb 1 Ascend

5 rounds
For time

## „WILLY"

- 800m Run
- 5 Front Squat 225lbs (100kg)
- 200m Run
- 11 Chest to Bar Pull-ups

- 400m Run
- 12 Kettlebell Swings (2 pood)

3 rounds
For time

## „COFFEY"

- 800m Run
- 50 Back Squat (M=135lbs – ca. 60kg, F=95lbs – ca. 40kg)
- 50 Bench Press (M=135lbs – ca. 60kg, F=95lbs – ca. 40kg)
- 800m Run
- 35 Back Squat (M=135lbs – ca. 60kg, F=95lbs – ca. 40kg)
- 35 Bench Press (M=135lbs – ca. 60kg, F=95lbs – ca. 40kg)
- 800m Run
- 20 Back Squat (M=135lbs – ca. 60kg, F=95lbs – ca. 40kg)
- 20 Bench Press, (M=135lbs – ca. 60kg, F=95lbs – ca. 40kg)
- 800m Run
- 1 Muscle-up

For time

## „TAYLOR"

- 400m Run
- 5 Burpee Muscle-ups

Use a weight vest if possible
4 rounds
For time

## „NUKES"

- 1 Mile Run
- Deadlifts max. reps 315lbs (ca. 60kg)
- Then, 10min to complete: 1 Mile Run and Power Cleans max. reps 225lbs (ca. 100kg)
- Then, 12min to complete: 1 Mile Run and Overhead Squats max. reps 135lbs (ca. 60kg)

No rest between the rounds
For time

## „ZEMBIEC"

- 11 Back Squats, 185lb (ca. 80kg)
- 7 Strict Burpee Pull-ups
- 400m Run

5 rounds
For time

# BODYWEIGHT

## „GI JANE"

100 Pull-up Burpees

For time

## „SEBW1"

- 50 Ring Dips
- 400m Run
- 50 Push-ups
- 400m Run
- 50 Handstand Push-ups
- 400m Run

For time

## „SEBW2"

- 21 Hip-Back Extensions
- 400m Run
- 18 Hip-Back Extensions
- 400m Run
- 15 Hip-Back Extensions
- 400m Run
- 12 Hip-Back Extensions
- 400m Run
- 9 Hip-Back Extensions
- 400m Run
- 6 Hip-Back Extensions
- 400m Run
- 3 Hip-Back Extensions

- 400m Run

For time

## „SEBW3"

- 1000m Row
- 25 Burpees
- 750m Row
- 50 Burpees
- 500m Row
- 75 Burpees

For time

## „SEBW4"

- 400m Run
- 15 Pull-ups
- 50 Squats
- 15 Pull-ups

3 rounds
For time

## „SEBW5"

- 400m Run
- 50 Squats
- 30 Back Extensions

5 rounds
For time

## „SEBW6"

- Row 250m
- 25 Push-ups

AMRAP: As Many Rounds As Possible in 15min

## „SEBW7"

- 100 Rope Jumps (Double Jump)
- 50 Push-ups
- 25 Pull-ups
- 1min L-Seat

For time

## „SEBW8"

- 10min Run
- 200 Squats
- 10min Run

For time

## „SEBW9"

- 50 Walking Lunges
- 50 Squats
- Run 400m

For time

## „SEBW10"

- 400m Run
- 25 Pull-ups
- 25 Push-ups
- 25 Crunches
- 25 Squats

For time

## „SEBW11"

- Tabata Sprints
- Tabata Squats

Maximum reps and distance
Tabata = 8x 20s/10s (Work/Rest)

## „SEBW12"

- 100 Jumping Jacks
- 100 Mountain Climbers

5 rounds
For time

## „SEBW13"

- 1000m Run
- 25 Push-ups
- 1000m Run

- 25 Air Squats
- 1000m Run
- 25 Pull-ups
- 1000m Run

For time

## „SEBW14"

- 100 Rope Jumps (Double Jumps)
- 100 Lunges
- 100 Rope Jumps (Alternate)
- 100 Squats

For time

## „SEBW15"

- Tabata Hill Sprints
- Tabata Push-ups
- Tabata Jumping Jacks
- Tabata Squats

Maximum reps

## „SEBW16"

- 200m Run
- 25 Push-ups

3 rounds
For time

## „SEBW17"

- 50 Burpees
- 75 Flutterkicks
- 100 Push-ups
- 150 Crunches

For time

## „SEBW18"

- 50 Pull-ups
- 400m Run
- 100 Push-ups
- 400m Run
- 150 Crunches
- 400m Run
- 200 Squats
- 400m Run
- 250 Double unders

For time

## „SEBW19"

- Pull-ups
- Squats Jumps
- Burpee

50-40-30-20-10 Repetitions
For time

## „SEBW20"

- Burpees
- Crunches

10-9-8-7-6-5-4-3-2-1 Repetitions
For time

## „SEBW21"

- 10 Lunge
- 10 Push-ups
- 50 Jumping Jacks

10 rounds
For time

## „SEBW22"

- 7 Muscle-ups
- 21 Burpees

5 rounds
For time

## „SEBW23"

- 7 Burpees
- 7 Crunches
- 7 Jumping Jacks

7 rounds
For time

## „SEBW24"

- 150 Push-ups
- 250 Burpees
- 500 Jumping Jacks

For time

## „SEBW25"

1000m Run and do every 100m:

- 5 Push-ups
- 10 Squats
- 20 Crunches

For time

# FREE WEIGHTS

## „SEFW1"

(115lbs = ca. 50kg)

- 500m Row
- 21 Push press 115lbs
- 500m Row
- 18 Push press 115lbs
- 500m Row
- 15 Push press 115lbs
- 500m Row
- 12 Push press 115lbs

For time

## „SEFW2"

- 15 Clean & Jerk 95lbs (ca. 45kg)
- 400m Run

AMRAP: As Many Rounds As Possible in 20min

## „SEFW3"

- 1 Deadlift (80% Bodyweight)
- 5 Power Snatches (80% Bodyweight)
- 15 Burpees

5 rounds
For time

## „SEFW4"

- 8 Front Squats (75% Bodyweight)
- 5 Weighted Pull-ups (25% Bodyweight)
- 100m Sprint

AMRAP: As many rounds as possible in 7min

## „SEFW5"

- 3 Squat clean
- 8 Toes to bar
- 6 Burpee box jumps

5 rounds
For time

## „SEFW6"

- 5 Deadlifts (100% Bodyweight)
- 10 Overhead Squats (50% Bodyweight)
- 15 Crunches
- 50 Jumping Jacks

AMRAP: As many rounds as possible in 10min

## „SEFW7"

- 8 Deadlift (100% Bodyweight)
- 50 Double unders
- 20 Benchpress (60% Bodyweight)

3 rounds
For time

## „SEFW8"

Use any weights

- 2 Hang power clean
- 3 Benchpress
- 4 Back Squats
- 5 Deadlifts

AMRAP: As many rounds as possible in 8min

## „SEFW9"

Use any weights

- 8 Deadlift
- 50 Double unders
- 100 High knees

3 rounds
For time

## „SEFW10"

- 7 Hang Squat Clean (Use any weights)
- 10 Clap Push-ups
- 30 Jumping Jacks

5 rounds
For time

## „SEFW11"

Use any weights

- 25 Thruster
- 25 Weighted Pull-ups
- 25 Benchpress
- 25 Sumo Deadlift High Pull
- 25 Burpees

For time

## „SEFW12"

Use any weights

- 3 Thruster
- 6 Burpee broad jumps

AMRAP: As many rounds as possible in 10min

## „SEFW13"

- 10 Overhead Squat (75% Bodyweight)
- 35 Double unders

5 rounds
For time

## „SEFW14"

- 1min Weighted Pull-ups (25% Bodyweight)

- 1min Benchpress (80% Bodyweight)
- 1min High knees

3 rounds
Maximum reps

## „SEFW15"

- 3 Deadlift (80% Bodyweight)
- 20 High Knees

AMRAP: As many rounds as possible in 9min

## „SEFW16"

Use any weights

- 3 Back Squats
- 5 Benchpress
- 7 Trap bar Deadlift

5 rounds
For time

## „SEFW17"

Use any weights

- Back Squat
- Ring Dips
- Burpee

21-15-9 Repetitions
For time

## „SEFW18"

Use any weights

- 3 Clean and Jerk
- 10 Ball Slams
- 25 High Knees

AMRAP: As many rounds as possible in 8min

## „SEFW19"

Use any weights

- 10 Pull-ups
- 10 Clean and Jerk
- 10 Box Jumps

3 rounds
For time

## „SEFW20"

- 3 Cluster
- 10 Jumping Jacks
- 5 Muscle-ups
- 20 High Knees

5 rounds
For time

## KETTLEBELL

Use kettlebells with every exercise, apart from the endurance exercises. Use any weights.

### „SEK1"

- Front Squat
- Bent Row
- Push-ups
- Burpee

22-16-10 Repetitions
For time

### „SEK2"

With 2 Kettlebells

- 10 Thruster
- 20 Snatch
- 30 Alternate Floor Press
- 40 Swing
- 50 Alternate Shoulder Press
- 40 Jumping Jacks
- 30 Step-up
- 20 Burpees

For time

### „SEK3"

- 3 Snatch (each Arm)
- 5 Burpee

AMRAP: as many rounds as possible in 20min

## „SEK4"

- 20 Burpee
- 18 Suitcase Deadlift
- 16 Push-ups
- 14 Clean
- 12 Pull-up (Kettlebell between the feet)
- 10 Push Press
- 100m Run-Sprint

2 rounds
For time

## „SEK5"

- Burpee with a Kettlebell
- 3 Back Squat
- 6 Double Kettlebell Swing
- 9 Push-ups

AMRAP: As many rounds as possible in 7min

## „SEK6"

- 5 Burpee
- 10 Swing
- 15 Bar dips (Kettlebell between the feet)
- 20 High knees

AMRAP: As many rounds as possible in 20min

## „SEK7"

- 60 Crunches (Kettlebell in hands)
- 50 Suitcase Deadlifts
- 40 Push-ups
- 30 Sumo High Pull
- 20 Burpee
- 10 Pistol Squats (one-leg Squats)
- 1000m Run

For time

## „SEK8"

- 10 Double Jerk
- 8 Snatch (each Arm)
- 5 Handstand Push-ups (on Kettelbells)
- 50 Jumping Jacks

5 rounds
For time

## „SEK9"

- 5 Benchpress
- 6 Burpees
- 7 Double Snatch
- 8 Jumping Jacks

5 rounds
For time

## „SEK10"

- Snatch 1-2-3-4-5-6 ... -14-15 Repetitions
- 400m Run
- Push-ups 15-14-13-12 ... -2-1 Repetitions
- 400m Run

For time

## „SEK11"

- 6 Snatch
- 12 Box Jumps (Kettlebell in hands)
- 18 Burpees

10 rounds
For time

## „SEK12"

- Snatch (alternating right and left)
- Handstand Push-up
- Burpees

21-15-9 Repetitions
For time

## „SEK13"

- 8 Single arm Thruster
- 8 Pistols (one-leg Squats)
- 8 Back Lunge
- 800m Run

8 rounds
For time

## „SEK14"

- 100 Swings
- 100 Goblet Squats
- 100 Burpees
- 100 Press
- 100 Suitcase Deadlift
- 100 Jumping Jacks
- 100 Thruster
- 100 High Knees

For time

## „SEK15"

- 20 Swing
- 30 Thruster
- 20 Push-ups
- 30 Crunches
- 20 Sumo Deadlift
- 30 Swing
- 20 Burpees (Kettlebell)

For time

## „SEK16"

- 50 Jumping Jacks
- 20 Swing
- 15 Push-up

- 10 Sumo Deadlift
- 5 Pistol (one-leg Squat)

5 rounds
For time

## „SEK17"

- 10 Snatch (alternating right and left)
- 10 Push-ups
- 50m Run-Sprint

AMRAP: As many rounds as possible in 10min

## „SK18"

- Clean and Jerk
- 1x10m Zonesprint - Run

1-2-3-2-3-4-3-4-5-4-5-6-5-6-7-6-7-8 Repetitions
For time

## „SEK19"

- 250 Swing
- 250 Burpees

For time

## „SEK20"

- 30 Front Squat

- 30 Push-ups
- 10 Snatch
- 10 Pull-ups (Kettlebell between the feet)
- 100 Rope Jumps (Double Jump)

3 rounds
For time

# MIXED

## „ANNIE ARE YOU OK?"

- 500m Row each Round
- Dumbbell Thruster 35lbs (ca. 15kg)
- Sumo-Deadlift High-Pull
- Burpees
- MedBall Clean 20lbs (ca. 8kg)
- Wallball 20lbs 10'

21-15-9 Repetitions
For time

## „FIGHT GONE BAD"

- Wallball 20lbs 10'
- Sumo-Deadlift to High-Pull 75lbs (ca. 30kg)
- Box Jump 24"
- Push Press 75lbs (ca. 30kg)
- Row (kcal)
- 1min Rest

3 or 5 rounds
For time

## „FILTHY FIFTY"

- 50 Box Jumps, 24"
- 50 Jumping Pull-ups
- 50 KB Swings 1 pood (apx 35lbs – ca. 15kg)
- Walking Lunges, 50 Steps
- 50 Knees to Elbows
- 50 Push Press, 45lb (ca. 20kg)

- 50 Back Extensions
- 50 Wallball, 20lb 10'
- 50 Burpees
- 50 Double Unders

For time

## „QUARTER GONE BAD"

- 15sec of: Thrusters 135lbs (ca. 60kg)
- 45s Rest
- 15s Weighted Pull-ups 50lbs (ca. 20kg)
- 45s Rest
- 15s Burpees
- 45s Rest

5 rounds
For time

## „SEM1"

- 400m Run
- 30 Overhead squats 75lbs (ca. 35kg)
- 21 Pull-ups

3 rounds
For time

## „SEM2"

- 15 Hang Power Snatch 95lbs (ca. 40kg)
- 400m Run

5 rounds
For time

## „SEM3"

- 25 Kettlebell swings 2 pood(70lbs – ca. 30kg)
- 25 GHD Sit-ups
- 25 Back Extensions
- 25 Knees to Elbows

5 rounds
For time

## „SEM4"

- 250m Row
- 21 Sumo-Deadlift High-Pull 95lbs (ca. 45kg)
- 15 Pull-ups

AMRAP: As Many Rounds As Possible in 20min

## „SEM5"

Use any weights

- 3 Power clean
- 4 Burpee Pull-ups

Every minute on the minute for 12min

## „SEM6"

Use any kettlebell

- 1 Double Kettlebell Snatch
- 1 Double Kettlebell Thruster
- 1 Burpees

Death by principle: Add on repetition for each exercise for every minute, till you can't do the necessary repetitions in one minute

## „SEM7"

Use any weight

- 5 Ground to overhead
- 5 Push-ups
- 10 Jumping Jacks

Every minute on the minute for 12min

## „SEM8"

Use any weights

- 400m Run
- 30 Ring Dips
- 30 Crunches
- 30 Thruster
- 30 Box Jumps
- 30 Kettlebell Swings
- 400m Run

For time

## „SEM9" –F.R.E.A.K.

Use any weights

- 21 Thruster
- 21 Pull-ups
- 800m Run
- 30 Kettlebell Swings
- 30 Pull-ups
- 50 Double unders
- 50 Crunches
- 400m Run
- 30 Box Jumps
- 30 Wall Balls
- 100m Sprint

For time

# „SEM10"

Use any weights

- 10 Muscle-ups
- 30 Kettlebell Swings
- 2min Row
- 60 Push Press
- 20 Push-ups
- 40 Kettlebell Swings
- 400m Run
- 100 Jumping Jacks
- 30 Crunches
- 15 Pull-up
- 50 Double Unders
- 10 Deadlifts

For time

## „SEM11"

- 100 Kettlebell Swings
- 400m Run
- 100 Kettlebell Goblet Squats
- 400m Run
- 100 Kettlebell Press
- 400m Run
- 100 Deadlifts (60% Bodyweight)
- 400m Run
- 100 Squats (60% Bodyweight)
- 400m Run

For time


## „SEM12"

- 50 Deadlifts (75% Bodyweight)
- 100 Pull-ups
- 200 Push-ups
- 300 Squats
- 400m Run
- 400m Run (backwards)

For time


## „SEM13"

Use any weights

- 10 Push Press
- 25 Push-ups
- 15 Hang Power clean
- 25 Pull-ups
- 20 Back Squats

- 25 Crunches
- 25 Deadlifts
- 25 Box Jumps
- 10m Row

For time

## „SEM14"

Use any weights

- 22 Deadlifts
- 200m Farmers Walk
- 22 Dumbbell Thrusters
- 200m Run
- 22 Pull-ups
- 400m Run
- 22 Overhead Squats
- 800m Run

For time

## „SEM15"

Use any weights

- 800m Run
- 60 Double unders
- 50 Back extensions
- 40 Crunches (use medicine ball or dumbbells)
- 30 Box Jumps
- 20 Deadlifts
- 10 Inverted Burpees
- 800m Run

For time

---

## „SEM16"

Use any weights

- 500m Row
- 100 Squats
- 400m Row
- 75 Push Press
- 300m Row
- 50 Deadlifts
- 200m Row
- 25 Kettlebell Swings

For time

---

## „SEM17"

Use any weights

- 25 Muscle-up
- 25 Deadlifts
- 25 Burpees
- 25 Pull-ups
- 25 Box Jumps
- 25 Ring Push-ups
- 25 Kettlebell Swings
- 25 Ring Dips
- 25 Double unders
- 25 Sumo Deadlifts
- 25x10m Sprint and 90m Walking

For time

## „SEM18"

Use any weights

- 10 Handstand Push-ups
- 20 Wall Ball
- 30 Toes to bar
- 40 Power clean
- 50 Burpees
- 60 Sumo Deadlift High Pull
- 100m Sled drag
- 100m Run-Sprint (back to start)

For time

## „SEM19"

Use any weights

- 3 Deadlifts
- 5 Box Jumps
- 10 High knees

Every minute on the minute for 10min

## „SEM20"

Use any weights

- 5 Burpees
- 1 Thruster
- 3 Pull-ups

Every minute on the minute for 12min

## OTHER WOD'S

### SLING TRAINER (E.G. TRX-SYSTEME)

Use a sling trainer with every exercise

„ST1"

- 25 Push-up
- 2min Rest

3 rounds
For time

„ST2"

- 25 Row
- 2min Rest

3 rounds
For time

„ST3"

40/40 Challenge

- Push-ups
- 60s Rest
- Row

Reach for 40 reps of each exercise

„ST4"

- 20 Jump Squat
- 10 Lunge (for every leg)

5 rounds
For time

## „ST5"

- 1min Plank
- 1min Mountain Climber
- 1min Plank
- 1min Rest

3 rounds

## „ST6"

- 10 Butterfly
- 10 Push-ups

5 rounds
For time

## „ST7"

- 10 Butterfly reverse
- 10 Row

5 rounds
For time

## „ST8"

- 25 Butterfly
- 25 Butterfly reverse

3 rounds
For time

## „ST9"

- 1 Butterfly
- 1 Row
- 1 Squat

Death by principle: Add on repetition for each exercise for every minute, till you can't do the necessary repetitions in one minute

## „ST10"

250 Push-ups

For time

## „ST11"

250 Row

For time

## „ST12"

500 Squats

For time

## „ST13"

- 5 Dips
- 5 Superman
- 5 Butterfly

5 rounds
For time

## „ST14"

- 100 Lunges
- 100 Push-ups
- 100 Butterfly reverse

For time

## „ST15"

- 10 one-arm Row (5 each side)
- 10 Squats

3 rounds
For time

## „ST16"

- 1min Backplank
- 1min Side Plank (left)

- 1min Plank
- 1min Side Plank (right)
- 1min Rest

3 rounds

## „ST17"

- 25 Side Lunge (left)
- 20 Row
- 25 Side Lunge (right)

2 rounds
For time

## „ST18"

- 10 Superman
- 10 Lunge (5 each side)

3 rounds
For time

## „ST19"

150 Superman

For time

## „ST20"

100 Dips

For time

---

„ST21"

- 1min Plank
- 30s Side Plank (each side)
- 30s Rest

5 rounds
For time

---

„ST22"

100 Pike Push

For time

---

„ST23"

50 One-arm row (each side)

For time

---

„ST24"

50 Handstand Push-ups (Use an appropriate angle)

For time

---

„ST25"

100 Plyo Squats

For time

# SPEED ROPES

## „SR1"

- 1min Double Jump
- 1min Rest

10 rounds
Maximum repetitions

## „SR2"

- 1min Alternate Jump
- 1min Rest

10 rounds
Maximum repetitions

## „SR3"

- 100 Double Jumps
- 10 Push-ups
- 20 Squats

3 rounds
For time

## „SR4"

20min Jump Rope with no rest

Maximum repetitions

## „SR5"

- 1min Double Jump (max. Speed)
- 1min Jump Rope (moderate speed)

6 rounds
Maximum repetitions

## „SR6"

- 10 Double Jumps
- 5 Push-ups
- 3 Pull-ups

AMRAP: As many rounds as possible in 15min

## „SR7"

- 50 Alternate Jumps
- 100m Run-Sprint
- 300m Run

4 rounds
For time

## „SR8"

- 50 Double Jumps
- 100m Swim (Freestyle)

4 rounds
For time

## „SR9"

- 10 Kettlebell Swing
- 100 Double Jumps

4 rounds
For time

## „SR10"

- 1min Double Jump
- 1min Alternate Jump

10 rounds
Maximum repetitions

## „SR11"

60min Jump Rope with rest as needed

Maximum repetitions

## „SR12"

- 1min Sky Jump
- 1min Rest

10 rounds
Maximum repetitions

## „SR13"

- 1min back and Forth Jump
- 1min Rest

10 rounds
Maximum repetitions

## „SR14"

- 1min Backwards Swing – Double Jump
- 1min Rest

10 rounds
Maximum repetitions

## „SR15"

- 1min Arms Cross Jump
- 1min Rest

10 rounds
Maximum repetitions

## „SR16"

- 1min max. Speed (Double Jump)
- 1min moderate Speed (Double Jump)

5 rounds
Maximum repetitions

## „SR17"

- 1min max. Speed (Alternate Jump)
- 1min moderate Speed (Alternate Jump)

5 rounds
Maximum repetitions

## „SR18"

- 1min max. Speed (Double Jump)
- 1min moderate Speed (Alternate Jump)

5 rounds
Maximum repetitions

## „SR19"

- 1min max. Speed (Alternate Jump)
- 1min max. Speed (Double Jump)
- 1min moderate Speed (Double Jump)

5 rounds
Maximum repetitions

## „SR20"

- 1min max. Speed (Alternate Jump)
- 1min max. (Double Jump)
- 1min moderate Speed (Alternate Jump)

5 rounds
Maximum repetitions

## AB-ROLLER

Use an AB-Whell or do a Barbell Rollout instead

**„AR1"**

10 AB-Rollouts

5 rounds
For time

**„AR2"**

- 100 AB-Rollouts
- 100 Crunches

For time

**„AR3"**

- 10 Side Rollouts (5 each side)
- 10 AB-Rollouts

3 rounds
For time

**„AR4"**

- 10 Burpees
- 10 AB-Rollouts
- 10 Push-ups

AMRAP: As many rounds as possible in 15min

## „AR5"

1 AB Rollout

Death by principle: Add on repetition for each exercise for every minute, till you can't do the necessary repetitions in one minute

## „AR6"

- 1min Plank
- 5 AB-Rollouts
- 10 Crunches

5 rounds
For time

## „AR7"

- 1 AB Rollout
- 1 Side Rollout (right)
- 1 Side Rollout (left)

AMRAP: As many rounds as possible in 10min

## „AR8"

- 10 Push-ups
- 5 Pull-ups
- 5 AB-Rollouts

8 rounds
For time

## „AR9"

- 50 Jumping Jacks
- 10 AB-Rollouts
- 50 High knees
- 10 AB-Rollouts

4 rounds
For time

## „AR10"

Learn a standing AB-Rollout

## „AR11"

Learn a one-handed Rollout

## „AR12"

- 10 Rollouts (hold 5s on toughest point)
- 1min Rest

4 rounds
For time

## „AR13"

- 5 Side Rollouts (rechts - hold 5s on toughest point)
- 1min Rest
- 5 Side Rollouts (links - hold 5s on toughest point)
- 1min Rest

3 rounds
For time


## „AR14"

- 5 Side Rollouts (rechts - hold 5s on toughest point)
- 1min Rest
- 5 Side Rollouts (links - hold 5s on toughest point)
- 1min Rest
- 10 Rollouts (gerade – hold 5s on toughest point)
- 1min Rest

3 rounds
For time


## „AR15"

- 10 Rollouts with a weight vest or a backpack with 10kg
- 1min Rest

3 rounds
For time

## CALISTHENICS CHALLENGES

Calisthenics is a training system that uses bodyweight exercises only. There are certain exercises that are really hard to master, so take your time and have patience with them.

„CC1"

Learn a Handstand

„CC2"

Learn a Human Flag

„CC3"

Learn a Pistol Squat

„CC4"

Learn a Headstand

„CC5"

Learn a Yoga-Scorpion

„CC6"

Learn a Dragon flag

„CC7"

Learn a one-arm Push-up

„CC8"

Learn a one-arm Pull-up

„CC9"

Learn a Front Lever

„CC10"

Learn a Back Lever

„CC11"

Learn a Flip

„CC12"

Learn a backflip

„CC13"

Learn a „Skin the cat"

## „CC14"

Learn a Handstand Walk

## „CC15"

Learn a Full Planche

## „CC16"

Learn a Nakayama

## „CC17"

Learn a Backbridge

## „CC18"

Learn a Muscle-up

## „CC19"

Learn a Crow Stand

„CC20"

**Learn a Crow to Handstand**

## CRAZY WOD'S

In this category you will find WOD'S which are very hard, some of them have to be completed within several days or even weeks or months.

## STRENGHT ONLY

„C1"

500 Push-ups

For time

„C2"

500 Pull-ups

For time

„C3"

1000 Push-ups in one week

„C4"

1000 Pull-ups in one week

„C5"

- 250 Push-ups
- 250 Pull-ups

- 250 Squats
- 250 Crunches

For time

## „C6"

- 1 Push-ups
- 1 Pull-up
- 1 Squat
- 1 Crunch

100 rounds
For time

## „C7"

1000 Squats in one day

## „C8"

100 Burpees on every day of a week

## „C9"

50 Push-ups every moring on 30 consecutive days

## „C10"

- 100 Push-ups
- 100 Pull-ups
- 100 Crunches
- 100 Squats

For time

## „C11"

500 Kettlebell Swing

For time

## „C12"

- 100 Benchpress
- 100 Barbell Row
- 100 Barbell Squat
- 5min Rest

2 rounds
For time

## „C13"

- 10 Box Jumps
- 10 Push-ups
- 10 Deadlifts
- 10 Kettlebell Clean and Jerk

20 rounds
For time

## "C14"

10.000 Crunches in one month

## "C15"

500 Kettlebell Thruster

For time

## "C16"

- 25 Barbell Overhead Squat
- 25 Kettlebell Deadlift
- 25 Box Jumps
- 3min Rest

10 rounds
For time

## "C17"

500 Barbell Push Press

For time

## "C18"

- 20 Push-ups
- 25 Crunches
- 20 Squats

Every morning on 30 consecutive days

## "C19"

10.000 Pull-ups in one year

## "C20"

10.000 Push-ups in one year

## "C21"

10.000 Crunches in one year

## "C22"

- 10 Push-ups
- 10 Benchpress

20 rounds
For time

## "C23"

- 10 Barbell Deadlift
- 10 Kettlebell Deadlift

20 rounds
For time

## „C24"

- 10 Barbell Row
- 10 Pull-ups

20 rounds
For time

## „C25"

- 100 Kettlebell Swing
- 100 Kettlebell Clean and Jerk
- 100 Kettlebell Deadlift
- 100 Kettlebell Push-ups
- 100 Kettlebell Squats

For time

## ENDURANCE ONLY

„C26"

Run a half marathon

„C27"

Run a marathon

„C28"

Run a ultra marathon

„C29"

Run a marathon in under 3 hours

„C30"

Run 100km in one week

„C31"

Run 100x100m Sprints in one week

„C32"

Run 1.000km in one year

„C33"

Run 10km every morning for one month

„C34"

500 Burpees

For time

„C35"

1000 Burpees in one week

„C36"

- 10 Burpees
- 10 Jumping Jack

20 rounds
For time

„C37"

- 5 Burpees
- 5 Jumping Jack

- 5 High knees

AMRAP: As many rounds as possible in 60min

---

„C38"

Do 100 Jumping Jacks every morning for one month

---

„C39"

Do 100 High knees every morning for one month

---

„C40"

5000m Schwimmen (Freestyle)

For time

---

„C41"

100km Bike

For time

---

„C42"

25km Row

For time

## "C43"

Do a Triathlon (Ironman distance)

For time

## "C44"

- 10km Run
- 100 Burpees
- 100km Bike

For time

## "C45"

Swim 50km in one month

## "C46"

Bike 500km in one month

## "C47"

1000m Swim (Breaststroke)

For time

## "C48"

- 1000m Swim (Breaststroke)
- 1000m Swim (Backstroke)
- 1000m Swim (Freestyle)

For time

## „C49"

Do 10.000km Endurance in one year (Bike/Swim/Run)

## „C50"

Run a marathon in every month of the year

## MORE CHALLENGES

- Combine every Crazy strenght and Endurance WOD to get hundreds of more WOD'S
- Try to do all the Crazy WOD'S in one year
- Find a partner and do all the Crazy WOD'S in one year together
- Repeat every regular WOD and try to beat your own results
- Learn a new kind of sport every year

## CREATING YOUR OWN WOD'S

To get thousands of more WOD'S you only have to follow this routine:

1. Choose a category (strenght/endurance/mixed)
2. Choose a method (AMRAP/Death by/For time)
3. Select your preferred exercises or use an existing WOD as a blueprint
4. Test your WOD
5. Implement it into your workout regimen if it works or fix it and go back to Step 4
6. Go back to Step 1

## LINKS

- www.roguefitness.com
- www.theboxmag.com
- www.woddrive.com

## EQUIPMENT

- Speedropes: Try Pro Speed Ropes
- Timer: Gymboss (on amazon)
- Affordable Equipment: www.badcompany.biz

Printed in Great Britain
by Amazon

44654399R00142